Swarm Intelligence and Evolutionary Algorithms in Healthcare and Drug Development

Swarm Intelligence and Evolutionary Algorithms in Healthcare and Drug Development

Edited by

Sandeep Kumar
Anand Nayyar
Anand Paul

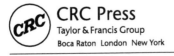

CRC Press
Taylor & Francis Group
Boca Raton London New York

CRC Press is an imprint of the
Taylor & Francis Group, an **Informa** business

A CHAPMAN & HALL BOOK

CRC Press
Taylor & Francis Group
52 Vanderbilt Avenue,
New York, NY 10017

© 2020 by Taylor & Francis Group, LLC

CRC Press is an imprint of Taylor & Francis Group, an Informa business

No claim to original U.S. Government works

Printed on acid-free paper

International Standard Book Number-13: 978-0-367-25757-6 (Hardback)

Visit the Taylor & Francis Web site at
http://www.taylorandfrancis.com

and the CRC Press Web site at
http://www.crcpress.com

Contents

Preface

The popularity of metaheuristics, especially swarm intelligence and evolutionary algorithms, has increased rapidly over the last two decades. Every year numerous algorithms and techniques are proposed by researchers, and progressively more novel applications are being found. When we think about our daily lives, we can sense that intelligent systems play more roles in our works or practical actions, and many differences have been observed in past few years in terms of intelligent approaches, methods and techniques. Currently, the field of metaheuristics, is impacting the scope of healthcare, especially in disease diagnosis and drug development.

Swarm intelligence has emerged as a new-generation methodology belonging to the class of evolutionary computing. While evolutionary computation, especially being biologically inspired, could be useful for the purpose of search and optimization, achieving the task of identifying an optimal solution out of a search place, typically vast and/or complex, and very much similar in line of natural evolution process. The underlying process of evolution is usually governed by some stochastic heuristic, applicable in a specific optimization context. In swarm intelligence, searching out an optimal in a search space is characterized by the way a swarm moves towards its goal. A swarm consists of number of particles, in which every one is engaged in the search process while on the move and maintains the best solution at any generation in the evolution in addition to the best reported by the entire swarm.

Applying swarm intelligence and evolutionary algorithms in healthcare and drug development is essential for the healthcare industry worldwide; this would continue to thrive and grow because diagnosis, treatment, disease prevention, medicine, and service affect the mortality rates and quality of life of human beings. Two key issues of the modern healthcare industry are improving healthcare quality, as well as reducing economic and human costs. The problems in the healthcare industry can be formulated as scheduling, planning, predicting, and optimization problems, where evolutionary computation methods can play a vital role. Although evolutionary computation has been applied to scheduling and planning for trauma systems and pharmaceutical manufacturing, other problems in the healthcare industry like decision-making in computer-aided diagnosis and predicting for disease prevention have not been properly formulated for evolutionary computation techniques, and many evolutionary computation techniques are not well known to the healthcare community.

The editors of this book were inspired to compile all swarm intelligence and evolutionary algorithms techniques and algorithms for healthcare, especially disease diagnosis and drug discovery, to provide readers to research on this potential avenue of optimization in more contexts.

The book would benefit several researchers and students as they can treat this as a strong base for exploring more opportunities of swarm intelligence and evolutionary algorithms in healthcare, and researchers can explore a lot of unexplored areas to find scope of problems to perform novel research.

The book has been categorized into six chapters to discuss applications of swarm intelligence and evolutionary computation in disease diagnosis especially for cancer, brain tumor, diabetic retinopathy and heart disease.

Chapter 1: **Swarm Intelligence and Evolutionary Algorithms in Disease Diagnosis—Introductory aspect** introduces basis of swarm and evolutionary algorithms. This chapter also discusses role of these algorithms in health care and detection of deadly diseases.

Chapter 2: **Swarm intelligence and Evolutionary Algorithms for Cancer Diagnosis** discusses various swarm intelligence as well as evolutionary algorithms that have been put forward in order to achieve fast diagnose of various forms of cancer. This chapter also discussed various stages and form of cancer.

Chapter 3: **Swarm Intelligence and Evolutionary Algorithms for Brain Tumor Diagnosis** discusses about diagnosis of brain tumor using nature inspired computing. Evolutionary and swarm intelligence are population-based optimization algorithms are prevalent optimization algorithms inspired by nature. The aim of this chapter is twofold, both discusses about brain tumor diagnosis. First, evolutionary algorithm and second, swarm intelligence algorithm. Here we present how to apply swarm intelligence and evolutionary algorithm for diagnosis of brain tumors.

Chapter 4: **Swarm Intelligence and Evolutionary Algorithms for Diabetic Retinopathy Detection** presents study of existing literature and tells about the different stages, features of diabetic retinopathy and the different types of models built to reduce the risk and early detection of diabetic retinopathy using evolutionary computing and swarm optimization.

Chapter 5: **Swarm Intelligence and Evolutionary Algorithms for Heart Disease Diagnosis** addresses heart disease diagnosis through swarm intelligence and evolutionary algorithms. First, the necessity of prediction and classification of heart disease using machine learning/swarm intelligence are addressed. Next, the diagnosis of coronary artery disease using the evolutionary algorithm. Then predicting heart attacks in patients using artificial intelligence methods are discussed. Further, swarm intelligence based optimization problem for heart disease diagnosis are presented. Finally, applying evolutionary algorithms for heart disease diagnosis are discussed.

Chapter 6: **Swarm Intelligence and Evolutionary Algorithms for Drug Design and Development** consists of a brief description of the need to predict molecular activity in the process of drug designing and monitoring over a body. Thereafter, it has briefly discussed the evolution and growth of the drug designing in the post and also elaborates the future aspects to look forward as an outcome of future discoveries. The next section deals about the role of swarm intelligence in the drug design as well as development process followed by evolutionary algorithms in the next section. In the later segments, the QSAR model has been discussed in context to cancer drug research. Finally, the chapter states the aspects of molecular activity prediction and the role of Swarm Intelligence and evolutionary algorithms for the same.

About the Editors

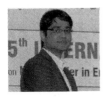 **Sandeep Kumar** is currently an Assistant Professor of Computer Science & Engineering at Amity University Rajasthan, Jaipur, India. Dr. Kumar holds a PhD degree in Computer Science & Engineering, M. Tech. degree from RTU, Kota, BE degree from Engineering College, Kota. Dr. Kumar was Assistant Professor of Computer Science & Engineering at ACEIT, Jaipur, 2008–2011, and Assistant Professor of Computer Science, Faculty of Engineering & Technology, Jagannath University, Jaipur, 2011–2017. Dr. Kumar was the head of computer science at Jagannath University, 2013–2017. He is also working as guest editor for special issue of many journals including *Int. J. of Intelligent Information and Database Systems (IJIIDS), Int. J. of Agricultural Resources, Governance and Ecology (IJARGE), Int. J. of Environment and Sustainable Development (IJESD), Inderscience, Recent Patents on Computer Science, Bentham Science*, and member of editorial boards for many international journals, and member of technical program committees of many conferences. He has delivered many keynote and expert talks in national/international conferences/workshop. He is also reviewer in many international journals and conferences, and acts as chairperson in many conferences. Dr. Kumar has over 50 publications in well-known SCI/SCOPUS indexed international journals and conferences, and has attended several national and international conferences and workshops. He has authored/edited four books in the area of computer science. His research interests include Nature Inspired Algorithms, Swarm Intelligence, Soft Computing and Computational Intelligence.

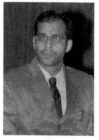

Anand Nayyar received a PhD degree in Computer Science from Desh Bhagat University in Mandi Gobindgarh. Currently, he is working as Lecturer, Researcher and Scientist at the Graduate School at Duy Tan University, Vietnam. He has 15+ years of academic teaching experience with more than 300 publications in reputed international conferences, journals and book chapters (indexed By: SCI, SCIE, Scopus, DBLP). Dr. Nayyar is a certified professional with more than 75 certifications from various IT companies like: CISCO, Microsoft, Oracle, Cyberoam, GAQM, Beingcert.com, ISQTB, EXIN, Google and many more. His areas of interest include: Wireless Sensor Networks, MANETS, Cloud Computing, Network Security, Swarm Intelligence, Machine Learning, Network Simulation, Ethical Hacking, Forensics, Internet of Things (IoT), Big Data, Linux and Open Source and Next Generation Wireless Communications. In addition, Dr. Nayyar is a Programme Committee Member/Technical Committee Member/Reviewer for more than 400 international conferences to date. He has published 30 books in Computer Science by various National and International Reputed Publishers like CRC Press, Elsevier, Springer, IGI-Global, BPB Publications, Scholar Press, GRIN etc. He has received 20 awards for teaching and research, including Young Scientist, Best Scientist, Exemplary Educationist, Young Researcher and Outstanding Reviewer Award. He is acting as Associate Editor of *IGI-Global Journal - International Journal of Information Security and Privacy (IJISP)*, *International Journal of Distributed Systems and Technologies (IJDST)*, *International Journal of Cognitive Informatics and Natural Intelligence* (IJCINI), and *International Journal of Green Computing (IJGC)*. He is acting as Editor-in-Chief of IGI-Global Journal "International Journal of Smart Vehicles and Smart Transportation (IJSVST)".

Anand Paul is currently working in The School of Computer Science and Engineering, Kyungpook National University, South Korea, as Associate Professor. He got his Ph.D. degree in electrical engineering at National Cheng Kung University, Taiwan, R.O.C., in 2010. His research interests include Algorithm and Architecture Reconfigurable Embedded Computing. He is a delegate representing South

Korea for M2M focus group and for MPEG. In 2004–2010 he has been awarded Outstanding International Student Scholarship, and in 2009, 2015 he won the best paper award in national computer Symposium, in Taipei, Taiwan, and international conference on Soft computing and network security, India.

He has guest-edited various international journals and he is also part of editorial team for *Journal of Platform Technology*. He serves as a reviewer for various *IEEE Transactions on Circuits and Systems for Video Technology*, *IEEE Transactions on System, Man and Cybernetics*, *IEEE Sensors*, *ACM Transactions on Embedded Computing Systems*, *IET Image Processing*, *IET Signal Processing* and *IET Circuits and Systems*. He gave invited talk in International Symposium on Embedded Technology workshop in 2012, He is the track chair for Smart human computer interaction in ACM SAC 2015, 2014. He is also an MPEG Delegate representing South Korea.

Contributors

Bhushan Inje
Department of Computer
  Engineering, SVKMs NMIMS
  (Deemed-to-be-University),
  Mukesh Patel School of
  Technology Management &
  Engineering, Shirpur, India

Sandeep Kumar
Department of Computer Science
  and Engineering
Amity University, Jaipur, India

Anand Nayyar
Graduate School
Duy Tan University, Da Nang,
  Viet Nam

Bandana Mahapatra
School of Mechnatronics
Symbiosis Skills and Open
  University, Pune, India

Dhananjay Joshi
Department of Computer
  Engineering, SVKMs NMIMS
(Deemed-to-be-University),
  Mukesh Patel School of
  Technology Management &
  Engineering, Shirpur, India

Nitin Choubey
Department of Information
  Technology, SVKM's NMIMS
  (Deemed-to-be-University),
  Mukesh Patel School of
  Technology Management &
  Engineering, Shirpur, India

Rajani Kumari
Department of Computer
  Application and IT
JECRC University, Jaipur

Sachin Bhandari
Department of Computer
  Engineering, SVKMs NMIMS
  (Deemed-to-be-University),
  Mukesh Patel School of
  Technology Management &
  Engineering, Shirpur, India

Radhakrishna Rambola
Department of Computer
  Engineering, SVKM's NMIMS
  (Deemed to be university),
  Mukesh Patel School of
  Technology Management &
  Engineering, Shirpur, India

Rajalakshmi Krishnamurthi
Department of Computer Science
Jaypee Institute of Information
  Technology, Noida, India

List of Abbreviations

SIEC	Swarm Intelligence and Evolutionary Computation
NIA	Nature Inspired Algorithms
SI	Swarm Intelligence
EA	Evolutionary Algorithms
PSO	Particle Swarm Optimization
MOECSA	Multi-Objective Ensemble Cuckoo Search Based on Decomposition
GA	Genetic Algorithm
PNN	Probabilistic Neural Network
DE	Differential Evolution
DBN	Dynamic Bayesian Network
EMO	Electromagnetism-like Optimization
EvoDM	Evolutionary Data Mining
FCM	Fuzzy C-Means
SWEET	Swarm, Evolutionary and Extraneous Topological Data Analysis
CAD	Computer-Aided Diagnosis
DR	Diabetic Retinopathy
NPDR	Non-proliferative Diabetic Retinopathy
PPDR	Pre-proliferative DR
IRMA	Intraretinal Microvascular Abnormalities
PDR	Proliferative Diabetic Retinopathy
NV	Neovascularization
NVD	Neovascularization Disc
MA	Microaneurysms
HEM	Haemorrhages
HE	Hard Exudates
SE	Soft Exudates

ME	Macular Edema
ANFIS	Adaptive Neuro Fuzzy Inference System
OCT	Optical Coherence Tomography
FAF	Fundus Auto-Fluorescence
GLCM	Gray-Level Co-occurrence Matrix
GBPD-RIS	Genetic-based Parameter Detector—Retinopathy Image - Segmentation
AMD	Age-Related Macular Degeneration
CRVO	Central Retinal Vein Occlusion
CNVO	Choroid Neo-vascularisation Membrane
CLBP	Complete Local Binary Pattern
HOG	Histogram of Oriented Gradient
ACO	Ant Colony Optimization
CVD	Cardio Vascular Diseases
CHD	Coronary Heart Disease
RHD	Rheumatic Heart Disease
CA	Cardiac Arrhythmias
CDSS	Clinical Decision Support System
MO-EOA	Multi-object Evolutionally Optimization Algorithm
LAD	Left Anterior Descending
RCA	Right Coronary Artery
LCX	Left Circumflex
ID3	Iterative Dichotomized 3
CART	Classification and Regression Tree
ADME	Absorption, Distribution, Metabolism and Excretion
CADD	Computer-Aided Drug Design
SBDM	Structure-Based Drug Design Method
LBDD	Ligand-Based Drug Design Method
HPC	High-Performance Computing Concept
BRGNN	Bayesian Regularised Genetic Neural Network
CIPN	Chemotherapy-Induced Peripheral Neuropathy
QSTR	Quantitative Structure Toxicity Relationship
QSAR	Quantitative Structure Activity Relationship
QSCR	Quantitative Structure Chromatography Relationships
QSTR	Quantitative Structure Toxicity Relationships
QSER	Quantitative Structure Electrochemistry Relationships
QSBR	Quantitative Structure Biodegradability Relationships
LWR	Locally Weighted Regression

Swarm Intelligence and Evolutionary Algorithms in Disease Diagnosis— Introductory Aspects

Bhushan Inje

Department of Computer Engineering, SVKM's NMIMS (Deemed-to-be-University), Mukesh Patel School of Technology Management & Engineering, Shirpur, India

Sandeep Kumar

Department of Computer Science and Engineering, Amity University, Jaipur, India

Anand Nayyar

Graduate School, Duy Tan University, Da Nang, Viet Nam

1.1 INTRODUCTION

Swarm intelligence and evolutionary computation (SIEC) are now very popular among researchers and scientists for the purpose of optimization. These approaches are also successful in health diagnosis and drug designing. The field of healthcare has large number of complex problems that are not solvable in polynomial time. The swarm intelligence and evolution computation techniques may be very helpful in prediction and diagnosis of deadly diseases. That is the main reason why medical scientists are trying to apply these approaches in clinical and biomedical areas.

The primary motivation of this study is to introduce the variety of SIEC techniques and algorithms that are being applied to healthcare and medicine to diagnose the diseases. SIEC provide help not only for doctors, counsellors and clinicians but also to them who play a technical role in the health industry, such as medical physicists, technicians and those who have an interest in learning more with a view to implementing systems or just understanding them better. Therefore, a brief overview of SIEC is required in various fields of healthcare and medicine for disease diagnosis, which has been provided in subsequent chapters of this book.

An overview of literature concentrating on the outstanding efforts by the authors is highlighted in Tables 1.1 and 1.2. These tables summarize various evolutionary algorithms proposed towards disease diagnosis and related research.

1.2 TERMINOLOGIES

1.2.1 Swarm Intelligence

Nature is always a source of inspiration as it offers the best solution to various complex problems efficiently and effectively without disturbing existing activities. Nature inspired algorithms (NIA) encouraged by some natural facts can be classified as per their source of inspiration. Major categories of NIA are the evolutionary algorithms and swarm algorithms. Swarm intelligence (SI) is the field of computational systems inspired by the collective intelligence of simple individual entities. Swarm intelligence is an emergent field of biologically adopted artificial intelligence motivated by the intelligent behaviour of insects, such as bees, wasps, ants and termites. Individually, these entities are not so intelligent but collectively they behave like an extraordinary single entity and work without any central control. This is possible due to the division of labour and the self-organizing behaviour. In 1988, researchers Gerardo Beni and Jing Wang introduced expression in the context of cellular robotic systems [1]. SI employ on a group of simple agents or birds communicating locally with others in the environment. The motivation frequently originates from nature, particularly biological systems. The best and popular examples are of bacterial growth, fish schooling, animal herding, microbial intelligence, bird flocking and ant colonies. These agents don't have centralized control structure over the behaviour, but they still interact with other agents. Major swarm intelligence-based algorithms are particle swarm optimization [2,34], artificial bee colony algorithm [3–6,29], spider monkey optimization algorithm [7,8], firefly algorithm [9,10] and many more.

Recently, large number of researchers and scientists are attracted towards these algorithms due to their simplicity, ease of implementation and very few control parameters. Literature shows that lots of research papers reported the successful use of SI-based algorithms in a wide range of applications, like structural optimization, scheduling, bioinformatics, machine learning, data mining, medical informatics, image analysis, industrial problems, operations research, dynamical systems and even finance and business. The applications of swarm intelligence are reported recently in robotics and mechatronics, popularly known as swarm robotics, while "swarm intelligence" is denoted as a universal set of algorithms. "Swarm prediction" is used in the applications like forecasting and predictions [17].

The potential of SI [12,22,37,41,42] is yet to be explored in many of the interesting application areas such as biomedical, bio-informatics and drug designing. There has been a slow growth reported in the past few years, as the number of methodologies proposed by the researchers that have successfully applied SI algorithms in field of biomedical is very less.

1.2.1.1 Merits of Swarm Intelligence

1. **Scalability**—These algorithms are applicable for wide range of problems. SI systems are highly scalable, as they are able to explore the complete solution search space, and it is interpreted as the control mechanisms are independent on swarm size.

2. **Adaptability**—These algorithms easily adapt the environmental conditions and try to converge into optimal solutions and react very quickly for varying surroundings and make use of self-organization capabilities and inherit auto-configuration. The adaptability permits them to adapt individual's behaviour to the environment at run-time basis, with wide-ranging flexibility.

3. **Cooperative robustness**—There is no central control in these algorithms and all the individuals work collectively because of its robust structure. However, the fault-tolerance skills are curiously high in SI systems, as all individuals communicate with others, therefore such systems don't have any chance of failure. The risk factor is reduced because the system works independently.

4. **Individual Simplicity**—The individual agents in swarm are very simple and not intelligent due to limited capabilities, but they collectively show intelligence.

The following four general principles are defined by Millonas in 1994 [14] regarding swarm intelligence:

1. **Proximity principle:** The basic elements of swarm must be able to perform simple computations with regard to their environment.

2. **Quality principle:** In addition to performing computations, swarms should comply with qualitative factors such as food and safe environment.

3. **Principle of diverse response:** This principle is concerned with the distribution of resources. The swarms should distribute the resources in an efficient manner for various nodes rather than a normal channel.

4. **Principle of stability and adaptability:** Swarms must be flexible enough to adapt to the changing environments and should change the modes without bearing high energy costs.

1.2.1.2 Classifications and Terminology

There are many ways to classify optimization algorithms; one of the most widely used is based on the quantity of agents, and another is based on the iteration procedure. The former will lead to two categories: single agent as well as multiple agents. Simulated annealing is considered as a single-agent algorithm with additional feature like a zigzag piecewise trajectory, whereas particle swarm optimization [2] and firefly algorithm [9] are population-based algorithms. These algorithms frequently have multiple agents with the interaction in a nonlinear manner, and a subset of which is called SI-based algorithm. For example, particle swarm optimization and firefly algorithm are swarm-based algorithms inspired by swarming behaviour of birds or fishes and fireflies, respectively.

Another way to classify algorithms is based on the core procedure of algorithms. If the procedure is fixed without any randomness, an algorithm that starts from a given initial value will reach the same final value, no matter how the algorithm is run. These algorithms are termed as "deterministic algorithms." For example, the classic Newton Raphson method is a deterministic algorithm and hill-climbing method is also deterministic. On the other hand, if an algorithm contains some randomness in the algorithmic procedure, then it is called "stochastic" or "heuristic" or even "metaheuristic." For example, genetic algorithms with mutation and crossover components can be called "evolutionary algorithms," "stochastic algorithms", or "metaheuristic algorithms." These different names for algorithms with stochastic components reflect an issue that there is still some confusion in the terminologies and terms used in the current literature. Algorithms, such as genetic algorithms, developed before 1980s were called "evolutionary algorithms," and now, they are termed as both evolutionary-based and metaheuristic [13,38]. Briefly speaking, heuristic means "trial and error," and metaheuristic can be considered a higher-level method by using certain information sharing and selection mechanisms. It is believed that the word "metaheuristic" was coined by Glover (1986) [16]. The multiple names and inconsistency in terminologies in the literature require efforts from research communities to agree on some of the common terminologies and to systematically classify and analyse algorithms.

1.2.2 Evolutionary Computation

Evolutionary computation (EC) is a collection of global optimization algorithms produced from artificial intelligence. The evolutionary computation techniques are implemented as key design elements in several computational models with evolutionary processes as problem-solving systems. Here evolution and optimization adopted from evolutionary concept in nature. On the basis of biological evolution, evolutionary computation solves the complex optimization problems. These techniques are widely used as analyser and prediction algorithms for healthcare applications. These types of techniques are used to solve the difficult problems like problem with large number of constraints or variables [16].

Darwinian theory says that the survival capability of the population may be improved by mutation in current population. According to some facts, higher chances of producing offspring is possible only for those individuals who live longer, in other words, genetic characters and their specific features are selected of the population. That's why the occurrences in evolutionary processes in various natural phenomena are emulated by computers, to convert these rules and apply these with the help of computation to enhance their ability towards knowledge gaining and design tools.

EC is a collection of various powerful techniques by following Darwinian evolution to achieve different functions such as optimization, learning and self-adaption.

1.2.3 Evolutionary Computation Paradigms

Evolutionary algorithms are based on the principle of "selection by nature," i.e. fittest individuals from current population will survive for next generation. Medical practitioners face lot of problems by logical thinking method while making critical decision over detection and diagnosis of a particular disease. Sometimes this complex approach leads the uncertainty and imprecision. This problem can be effectively solved by the means of intelligent decision-making systems using NIA. According to Darwin [15], evolutionary algorithms (EAs) are computational intelligence techniques that are inspired by the basic concept of evolution in nature, such as competition, variation, probability of survival, inheritance and reproduction. EAs make quality criteria or rules to work and use these rules to compare the population and to measure candidate solutions [17–18].

These algorithms use some operators analogous to natural process, such as mutation, crossover and selection. The selection operator denotes a process to select best individuals for mating with good chances of survival and suitable for competition. Mutation and reproductions are two main variation operators in EAs inspired by natural biological process of reproduction and gene mutation. Small changes in the part of an individual's structure are referred to as mutation, and this exchange some features of an individual to create descendants by the combination of their parents. It concludes that due to mutation some new offspring were introduced as new genetic material into the population.

Figure 1.1 shows the process for computation of fitness, in EAs fitness of a solution decides its quality, or it is also known as survival probability for an individual. The fitness function is measured by an algebraic function using value of function, and this process of fitness calculation is referred to as evaluation of individuals. If fitness of an individual is computed directly, then it is known as "phenotype" and its exact opposite operation is termed as "genotype," which represents the decoding of synthetic structure for an individual analogous to DNA coding

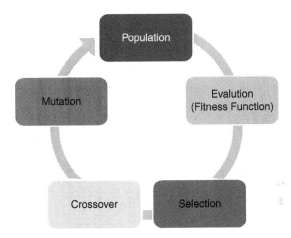

FIGURE 1.1   Process for fitness function.

of living beings. It obviously represents that in nature, recombination, mutation and inheritance act as genotype, whereas selection acts as phenotype in EAs.

1.3 IMPORTANCE OF SWARM INTELLIGENCE IN DISEASE DIAGNOSIS

Large number of researchers and practitioners recently utilized computational intelligence for diagnosing varied diseases. All these techniques are helpful for general practitioners to diagnose diseases with very less chances of failure.

Kumar et al. [17] discussed importance of artificial bee colony algorithm, firefly algorithm and bat algorithm in the field of healthcare. These algorithms are getting the attention of researchers rapidly, while they are comparatively new in the area of swarm intelligence. This is happening because of their ease of implementation and simplicity. Population-based nature-inspired algorithms have applications in nearly every single field, including computer science; engineering; mathematics; energy; agricultural sciences; biological sciences; physics; astronomy; biochemistry; molecular biology; genetics; material sciences; environmental sciences; business, management and accounting; social sciences; and medical sciences, among others.

Swarm intelligence techniques are considered as problem-solving techniques that are developed in the interactions of simple information processing task. The information processing task arranged as swarm can be animated, machine-driven, computational, or scientific; can be insects, birds, or human beings; can be robots or standalone workstations, and can be real or imaginary. Their joins can have a wide range of character-istics, but there must be proper collaboration among the individuals. This phenomenon is known as "swarm intelligence."

Correct and timely disease diagnosis is one of the most important challenges in medicine. There are many applications in the area of healthcare and disease diagnosis, some of which are enlisted in the subsequent paragraphs.

Abdullah and Selvakumar [19] discussed leading cause for death and disability as type II diabetes, which is considered as one of the prolonged diseases in most of the countries. The aim of this research is to apply improved PSO with decision tree for retrieving the risk factors for type II diabetes. They used normal and abnormal levels to denote the parameters for type II diabetes to understand the risk. Researchers suggested enhanced combination of PSO using decision trees along with different splitting measures with real-world diabetic dataset. With enhanced PSO, self-adaptive inertia weight with modified convergence logic for particles is used to accelerate in the given search space. As per results, there are various parameters or factors on which severity of diabetes can be measured, such as post-prandial plasma glucose (PPG), mean blood glucose (MBG), glycosylated haemoglobin (A1c) and fasting plasma glucose (FPG) were identified with an improved accuracy more than that of the existing methods and algorithms. Fisher's linear dis-criminant analysis is used to test efficiency of prediction. From the interpretation they argue that the risk factors have strong relationship, such as PPG, A1c, MBG and FPG with the risk corresponding to type II diabetes. Hence, in order to identify risk factors corresponding to other chronic diseases such as coronary heart disease and kidney disease, predictive analytics using an enhanced improved PSO using decision trees can also be deployed.

Rani and Ramyachitra [20] used swarm intelligence for cancer gene selection and classification. The work focussed on two objectives i.e. Cancer gene feature selection by using spider monkey optimization algorithm to eliminate irrelevant and redundant genes and support vector machine classification algorithm for classification of microarray cancer gene expression data. The proposed method has experimented

TABLE 1.1 Swarm Intelligence in Disease Diagnosis

Sr. No.	Disease Name	Title of Paper	Author Name	Applied Algorithms
1.	Breast cancer	Swarm Intelligence Approach for Breast Cancer Diagnosis [35]	Hoda Zamani, Mohammad-Hossein Nadimi-Shahraki	PSO, ICA, FA and IWO
2.	Hepatitis	Research Article on Hepatitis Disease Diagnosis Using Hybrid Case Based Reasoning and Particle Swarm Optimization [27]	Mehdi Neshat, Mehdi Sargolzaei, Adel Nadjaran Toosi, and Azra Masoumi	PSO and CBR
3.	Breast cancer	Computer-Aided Detection of Breast Cancer on Mammograms: A Swarm Intelligence Optimized Wavelet Neural Network Approach [28]	J. Dheeba, N. Albert Singh, S. Tamil Selvi	Particle Swarm Optimized Wavelet Neural Network (PSOWNN)
4.	Type II diabetes	Assessment of the Risk Factors for Type II Diabetes Using an Improved Combination of Particle Swarm Optimization and Decision Trees by Evaluation with Fisher's Linear Discriminant Analysis [19]	A. Sheik Abdullah S. Selvakumar	Particle swarm optimization, decision trees and Fisher's linear discriminant analysis
5.	Cancer subtype	Nature-Inspired Multi-Objective Cancer Subtype Diagnosis [30]	Yunhe Wang, Bo Liu, Zhiqiang Ma, Ka-Chun Wong, and Xiangtao Li	Multi-objective ensemble cuckoo search based on decomposition (MOECSA)
6.	Cancer	Microarray Cancer Gene Feature Selection Using Spider Monkey Optimization Algorithm and Cancer Classification Using SVM [20]	R. Ranjani Rani, D. Ramyachitra	Spider Monkey Optimization Algorithm, SVM

(Continued)

TABLE 1.1 (Cont.)

Sr. No.	Disease Name	Title of Paper	Author Name	Applied Algorithms
7.	Breast cancer	Missing Value Imputation for Breast Cancer Diagnosis Data Using Tensor Factorization Improved by Enhanced Reduced Adaptive Particle Swarm Optimization [21]	Atefeh Nekouie, Mohammad Hossein Moattar	Modified tensor factorization method, particle swarm optimization algorithm with adaptive adjustment (RAPSO)
8.	Chronic hepatitis C	Comparison of Machine Learning Approaches for Prediction of Advanced Liver Fibrosis in Chronic Hepatitis C Patients [11]	Somaya Hashem, Gamal Esmat, Wafaa Elakel, Shahira Habashy, Mohamed Elhefnawi, Mohamed I. Eladawy, Mahmoud ElHefnawi	Particle swarm optimization, decision tree, multi-linear regression and genetic algorithm
9.	Skin cancer	Intelligent Skin Cancer Detection Using Enhanced Particle Swarm Optimization [43]	Teck Yan Tan, Li Zhang, Siew Chin Neoh, Chee Peng Lim	Dermoscopic images using a variant of the Particle Swarm Optimization (PSO) algorithm
10.	Parkinson's disease	A New Hybrid Intelligent Framework for Predicting Parkinson's Disease [23]	Z. Cai, J. Gu and H. Chen	Support vector machine (SVM) based on bacterial foraging optimization (BFO)

with various benchmark cancer datasets and it reveals that the proposed method outperforms all other existing techniques in terms of the minimum number of features and maximum classification accuracy.

1.4 IMPORTANCE OF EVOLUTIONARY ALGORITHMS IN DISEASE DIAGNOSIS

Recently, healthcare professionals have faced problems with regard to the large amounts of medical data available for heterogeneous disease test cases, for example, cancer, heart diseases, etc.

Cancer is a group of associated diseases in which some of the body's cells begin to divide without stopping and spread into surrounding tissues. Nowadays, heart diseases and cancer are universal cause of human death. This leads to tons of challenges for healthcare professionals. Some well-known medical institutes provide medical datasets for the purpose of research to detect these deadly diseases in the early stage and to speed up the diagnosis process. According to Table 1.2, evolutionary algorithms not only solve these challenges but also help to overcome various problems faced by professionals via traditional approaches.

Many opportunities are available for cancer diagnosis research. Cancer diagnosis has long relied on the microscopic examination of cells to find the appearance of cancer cells. Other opportunities lie in finding new and better tools for imaging tumours from different samples or test cases. Major challenges are encountered in diagnostic tests, where results must be reliable and also returned to patients and doctors within a relatively short time frame. There are some common cancer types like bladder cancer, breast cancer, colorectal cancer, kidney (renal cell) cancer, leukaemia, liver cancer, lung cancer, lymphoma, pancreatic cancer, prostate cancer, skin cancer, thyroid cancer, uterine cancer, etc. These types of cancers are commonly detected and are the main cause of increased human death rate [32,33].

Dimitrios Mantzaris et al. [25] depict a variant of genetic algorithms to create subgroups of patients' information that is used as an input for probabilistic neural networks (PNNs). After reasonable steps of genetic evolution, the GA congregated to diagnostic factors subgroups that were consisted from some diagnostic factors. The proposed advanced PNNs outperformed the full-trained PNNs in terms of the MSE. Therefore, the implementation of PNNs is based on some precisely selected diagnostic factors, that resulted not only in the increase of PNNs' performance and predictive ability but also the training procedure was accelerated. The final conclusion needs to be drawn in this way because the number of diagnostic factors for appendicitis prediction may be filtered with no negotiation to the fidelity of clinical evaluation.

There is new variation of Differential Evolution (DE) algorithm being implemented by Akutekwe et al. [26]. A novel algorithm is proposed that outperformed various methods of the support vector machine (SVM). Wilcoxon rank-based sum test method is applied and presented in a manner, that there is momentous variation between the performances of the different DE algorithms, while some variants had similar performances based on their p-values. Researchers argued that DE/best/2 has best performance on SVM-Radial algorithm, which selected few high-quality features using the average best solution values.

Biji and Hariharan [24] presented an algorithm for the detection of white blood cells using smear images that considered the investigation of circle detection problem. The approach is referred to a nature-inspired technique called the "electromagnetism-like optimization (EMO) algorithm." This algorithm is a heuristic method that works on electromagnetism principles to solve composite optimization problems. The technique is validated using images of blood cells with different complexity range and the efficiency of the technique checked by robustness and stability.

TABLE 1.2   Evolutionary Algorithms in Disease Diagnosis

Sr. No.	Disease Name	Title of Paper	Author Name	Applied Algorithms
1.	Hepatocellular carcinoma (liver cancer)	An Optimized Hybrid Dynamic Bayesian Network Approach using Differential Evolution Algorithm for the Diagnosis of Hepatocellular Carcinoma [26]	A. Akutekwe, H. Seker and S. Iliya	Differential Evolution algorithm, Dynamic Bayesian Network (DBN)
2.	Acute leukaemia	An Efficient Peripheral Blood Smear Image Analysis Technique for Leukaemia Detection [24]	G. Biji and S. Hariharan	Electromagnetism-like optimization (EMO)
3.	Medical disease prediction	An Evolutionary Technique for Medical Diagnostic Risk Factor Selection [25]	Dimitrios Mantzaris, George Anastassopoulos, Lazaros Iliadis, Adam Adamopoulos	Probabilistic Neural Networks (PNNs), Genetic Algorithm (GA)

(Continued)

TABLE 1.2   (Cont.)

Sr. No.	Disease Name	Title of Paper	Author Name	Applied Algorithms
4.	Prostate cancer	A Survey on Computational Intelligence Approaches for Predictive Modelling in Prostate Cancer [36]	Georgina Cosma, David Brown, Matthew Archer, Masood Khan, A. Graham Pockley	Computational Intelligence
5.	Cardiac disease	Development of Evolutionary Data Mining Algorithms and Their Applications to Cardiac Disease Diagnosis [18]	Jenn-Long Liu; Yu-Tzu Hsu; Chih-Lung Hung	Evolutionary data mining (EvoDM) algorithms, Momentum-type particle swarm optimization (MPSO) and K-means algorithm
6.	Cardiovascular heart disease	Improving the Heart Disease Diagnosis by Evolutionary Algorithm of PSO and Feed Forward Neural Network [44]	Majid Ghonji Feshki, Omid Sojoodi Shijani	Particle Swarm Optimization, Neural Network Feed Forward Backpropagation
7.	Heart disease	Using PSO Algorithm for Producing Best Rules in Diagnosis of Heart Disease [39]	Azhar Hussein Alkeshuosh, Mariam Zomorodi Moghadam, Inas Al Mansoori, Moloud Abdar	Particle Swarm Optimization (PSO)
8.	Liver Cirrhosis Disease	Evolutionary Feature Construction for Ultrasound Image Processing and its Application to Automatic Liver Disease Diagnosis [31]	Yu-Hsiang Wu, Jhu-Yun Huang, Shyi-Chyi Cheng, Chen-Kuei Yang, Chih-Lang Lin	Evolutionary feature construction
9.	Hepatic cancer	An Evolutionary Computational Approach to Probabilistic Neural Network with Application to	F. Gorunescu, M. Gorunescu, E. El-Darzim, S. Gorunescu	Probabilistic Neural Networks, Evolutionary computational approach

(Continued)

TABLE 1.2   (Cont.)

Sr. No.	Disease Name	Title of Paper	Author Name	Applied Algorithms
		Hepatic Cancer Diagnosis [40]		
10.	Breast cancer	Analytics of Heterogeneous Breast Cancer Data Using Neuro-evolution [32]	Beibit Abdikenov, Zangir Iklassov, Askhat Sharipov, Shahid Hussain, Prashant K. Jamwal	Deep neural networks (DNNs)
11.	Diabetic retinopathy	Automatic Detection of Retinal Lesions for Screening of Diabetic Retinopathy [33]	Sudeshna Sil Kar, Santi P. Maity	Differential evolution algorithm

In growth of evolutionary data mining algorithms and their applications to cardiac disease diagnosis, Liu et al. [18] contributed for cardiac disease prediction and introduced two variation of EvoDM algorithms. Two cardiac disease datasets were studied for training purpose and improving the strength of algorithm. From their results they concluded that by using two EvoDM algorithms it achieved excellent enhancement in clustering accuracy and also received help during diagnosis of cardiac disease.

1.5 CONCLUSION

Swarm intelligence and evolutionary algorithms that are used for disease diagnosis have been discussed in this chapter. Many researchers proposed state-of-art techniques and hybrid approaches to achieve optimum results in different healthcare applications. Some of the techniques are prune to reduce the time complexity as well as the feature reduction in the classification problems. There are many medical application areas for these algorithms like cancer diagnosis, brain tumour diagnosis, diabetic retinopathy detection, heart disease diagnosis and drug design and development in healthcare industries. This chapter focuses on the implementation of swarm intelligence and evolutionary algorithms in the field of healthcare and drug designing. According to literature, it has been observed that many techniques have been proposed recently for automated process of diagnosis of various diseases.

REFERENCES

1. G. Beni (1988, August 24–26).Concept of Cellular Robotic Systems. In: Presented at the 3rd IEEE Symposium on Intelligent Control. Arlington, Virginia.
2. J. Kennedy, & R. Eberhart (1995). Particle Swarm Optimization. In: Proceedings of the IEEE international conference on neural networks (vol. 4, pp. 1942–1948). IEEE.
3. D. Karaboga, (2005). An Idea based on Honey Bee Swarm for Numerical Optimization. Technical Report TR06, Erciyes University, Engineering Faculty, Computer Engineering Department.
4. Nayyar A., Puri V., Suseendran G. (2019) Artificial Bee Colony Optimization—Population-Based Meta-Heuristic Swarm Intelligence Technique. In: Balas V., Sharma N., Chakrabarti A. (eds) Data Management, Analytics and Innovation. Advances in Intelligent Systems and Computing, vol 839. Springer, Singapore.
5. J. C. Bansal, H. Sharma, & S. S. Jadon (2013). Artificial Bee Colony Algorithm: A Survey. International Journal of Advanced Intelligence Paradigms, 5(1–2), 123–159.
6. S. Sharma, S. Kumar, & A. Nayyar (2018, August). Logarithmic Spiral Based Local Search in Artificial Bee Colony Algorithm. In: International Conference on Industrial Networks and Intelligent Systems (pp. 15–27). Springer, Cham.
7. J. C. Bansal, H. Sharma, S. S. Jadon, & M. Clerc (2014). Spider Monkey Optimization Algorithm for Numerical Optimization. Memetic Computing, 6(1), 31–47.
8. S. Kumar, A. Nayyar, N. G. Nguyen, & R. Kumari (2019). Hyperbolic Spider Monkey Optimization Algorithm. Recent Patents on Computer Science, 12 (1). doi:10.2174/2213275912666181207155334.
9. X. S. Yang (2009, October). Firefly Algorithms for Multimodal Optimization. In: International Symposium on Stochastic Algorithms (pp. 169–178). Springer, Berlin, Heidelberg.
10. Durbhaka G.K., Selvaraj B., Nayyar A. (2019) Firefly Swarm: Metaheuristic Swarm Intelligence Technique for Mathematical Optimization. In: Balas V., Sharma N., Chakrabarti A. (eds) Data Management, Analytics and Innovation. Advances in Intelligent Systems and Computing, vol 839. Springer, Singapore.
11. S. Hashem et al. (2018, May-June 1). Comparison of Machine Learning Approaches for Prediction of Advanced Liver Fibrosis in Chronic Hepatitis C Patients. IEEE/ACM Transactions on Computational Biology and Bioinformatics, 15(3),861–868. doi:10.1109/TCBB.2017.2690848.
12. M. Belal, J. Gaber, H. El-Sayed, & A. Almojel (2006). Swarm Intelligence, In Handbook of Bioinspired Algorithms and Applications. Series: CRC

Computer & Information Science, 7, Chapman & Hall Eds, (pp 4-55-4-62), ISBN 1-58488-477-5.

13. A. Nayyar, & R. Singh (2016). Ant Colony Optimization - Computational swarm intelligence technique. In: 2016 3rd International Conference on Computing for Sustainable Global Development (INDIACom) (pp. 1493–1499), Bharati Vidyapeeth's Institute of Computer Applications and Management (BVICAM). New Delhi.

14. M. Millonas. Swarms, Phase Transitions, and Collective Intelligence. Addison-WesleyPublishing Company, Reading (1994).

15. P. Acot (1983). Darwin et l'écologie. Revue d'Histoire des Sciences, 36, 33–48.

16. F. Glover (1986). Future Paths for Integer Programming and Links to Artificial Intelligence. Computers & OR, 13, 533–549.

17. K. Sandeep, & R. Kumari (2018). Artificial Bee Colony, Firefly Swarm Optimization, and Bat Algorithms. In: Nguyen Gia Nhu, Anand Nayyar, Dac-Nhuong Le (Lê Đắc Nhường), Advances in Swarm Intelligence for Optimizing Problems in Computer Science (pp. 145–182). Chapman and Hall/CRC.

18. J. Liu, Y.-T. Hsu, & C.-L. Hung (2012). Development of Evolutionary Data Mining Algorithms and their Applications to Cardiac Disease Diagnosis. In: 2012 IEEE Congress on Evolutionary Computation (pp. 1–8). Brisbane, QLD. doi: 10.1109/CEC.2012.6256640.

19. A. Sheik Abdullah, & S. Selvakumar. Assessment of the Risk Factors for Type II Diabetes Using an Improved Combination of Particle Swarm Optimization and Decision Trees by Evaluation with Fisher's Linear Discriminant Analysis. S. Soft Comput (2018). Springer Berlin Heidelberg, https://doi.org/10.1007/s00500-018-3555-5

20. R. Ranjani Rani, & D. Ramyachitra (2018). Microarray Cancer Gene Feature Selection Using Spider Monkey Optimization Algorithm and Cancer Classification Using SVM. Procedia Computer Science, 143, 108–116, ISSN 1877-0509. doi:10.1016/j.procs.2018.10.358.

21. A. Nekouie, & M. H. Moattar (2018). Missing Value Imputation for Breast Cancer Diagnosis Data using Tensor Factorization Improved by Enhanced Reduced Adaptive Particle Swarm Optimization. Journal of King Saud University – Computer and Information Sciences, ISSN 1319-1578. doi;10.1016/j.jksuci.2018.01.006.

22. A. Nayyar, & N. G. Nguyen (2018). Introduction to Swarm Intelligence. In: Anand Nayyar, Dac-Nhuong Le, Nhu Gia Nguyen, Advances in Swarm Intelligence for Optimizing Problems in Computer Science (pp. 53–78). Chapman and Hall/CRC.

23. Z. Cai, J. Gu, & H. Chen (2017). A New Hybrid Intelligent Framework for Predicting Parkinson's Disease. IEEE Access, 5, 17188–17200. doi:10.1109/ACCESS.2017.2741521.

24. G. Biji, & S. Hariharan (2017). An Efficient Peripheral Blood Smear Image Analysis Technique for Leukemia Detection. In: 2017 International Conference on I-SMAC (IoT in Social, Mobile, Analytics and Cloud) (I-SMAC) (pp. 259–264). Palladam. doi: 10.1109/I-SMAC.2017.8058350.

25. D. Mantzaris, G. Anastassopoulos, L. Iliadis, & A. Adamopoulos (2009). An Evolutionary Technique for Medical Diagnostic Risk Factors Selection. In: Iliadis, L., Vlahavas, I., & Bramer, M. (Eds.), IFIP International Federation for Information Processing, Volume 296; Artificial Intelligence Applications and Innovations III (pp. 195–203). Boston: Springer.

26. A. Akutekwe, H. Seker, & S. Iliya (2014). An Optimized Hybrid Dynamic Bayesian Network Approach Using Differential Evolution Algorithm for the Diagnosis of Hepatocellular Carcinoma. In: 2014 IEEE 6th International Conference on Adaptive Science & Technology (ICAST) (pp. 1–6). Ota. doi: 10.1109/ICASTECH.2014.7068140.

27. Mehdi Neshat, Mehdi Sargolzaei, Adel Nadjaran Toosi, and Azra Masoumi (2012), "Hepatitis Disease Diagnosis Using Hybrid Case Based Reasoning and Particle Swarm Optimization," ISRN Artificial Intelligence, vol. 2012, Article ID 609718, 6 pages. https://doi.org/10.5402/2012/609718.

28. J. Dheeba, N. Albert Singh, & S. Tamil Selvi (2014). Computer-Aided Detection of Breast Cancer on Mammograms: A Swarm Intelligence Optimized Wavelet Neural Network Approach. Journal of Biomedical Informatics, 49, 45–52, ISSN 1532-0464. doi:10.1016/j.jbi.2014.01.010.

29. S. Kumar, A. Nayyar, & R. Kumari (2019). Arrhenius Artificial Bee Colony Algorithm. In: Bhattacharyya, S., Hassanien, A., Gupta, D., Khanna, A., & Pan, I. (Eds.), International Conference on Innovative Computing and Communications. Lecture Notes in Networks and Systems, Vol. 56. Pages 187–195, Springer, Singapore.

30. Y. Wang, B. Liu, Z. Ma, K. Wong, & X. Li. (2019). Nature-Inspired Multiobjective Cancer Subtype Diagnosis. IEEE Journal of Translational Engineering in Health and Medicine, 7, 1–12, Art no. 4300112. doi:10.1109/JTEHM.2019.2891746.

31. Y. Wu, J. Huang, S. Cheng, C. Yang, & C. Lin (2011). Evolutionary Feature Construction for Ultrasound Image Processing and its Application to Automatic Liver Disease Diagnosis. In: 2011 International Conference on Complex, Intelligent, and Software Intensive Systems (pp. 565–570). Seoul. doi: 10.1109/CISIS.2011.93.

32. B. Abdikenov, Z. Iklassov, A. Sharipov, S. Hussain, & P. K. Jamwal (2019). Analytics of Heterogeneous Breast Cancer Data Using Neuro evolution. IEEE Access, 7, 18050–18060. doi:10.1109/ACCESS.2019.2897078.

33. S. S. Kar, & S. P. Maity (2018). Automatic Detection of Retinal Lesions for Screening of Diabetic Retinopathy. IEEE Transactions on Biomedical Engineering, 65(3),608–618, March. doi:10.1109/TBME.2017.2707578.

34. P. Bhambu, S. Kumar, & K. Sharma (2018). Self Balanced Particle Swarm Optimization. International Journal of System Assurance Engineering and Management, 9(4), 774–783.

35. H. Zamani, & M.-H. Nadimi-Shahraki (2016, October). Swarm Intelligence Approach for Breast Cancer Diagnosis. International Journal of Computer Applications Vol151(1). Pages (0975–8887).

36. G. Cosma, D. Brown, M. Archer, A. Masood Khan, & G. Pockley (2017). A Survey On Computational Intelligence Approaches for Predictive Modelling in Prostate Cancer. Expert Systems with Applications, 70, 1–19, ISSN 0957-4174. doi:10.1016/j.eswa.2016.11.006.

37. A. Nayyar, S. Garg, D. Gupta, & A. Khanna (2018). Evolutionary computation: Theory and algorithms. In: Anand Nayyar, Dac-Nhuong Le, Nhu Gia Nguyen, Advances in Swarm Intelligence for Optimizing Problems in Computer Science (pp. 1–26). Chapman and Hall/CRC.

38. Mirjalili, S. (2019). Genetic algorithm. In Evolutionary Algorithms and Neural Networks (pp. 43–55). Springer, Cham.

39. A. H. Alkeshuosh, M. Z. Moghadam, I. A. Mansoori, & M. Abdar (2017). Using PSO Algorithm for Producing Best Rules in Diagnosis of Heart Disease. In: 2017 International Conference on Computer and Applications (ICCA) (pp. 306–311). Doha. doi: 10.1109/COMAPP.2017.8079784.

40. F. Gorunescu, M. Gorunescu, E. El-Darzi, & S. Gorunescu (2005). An Evolutionary Computational Approach to Probabilistic Neural Network with Application to Hepatic Cancer Diagnosis. In: 18th IEEE Symposium on Computer-Based Medical Systems (CBMS'05) (pp. 461–466). Dublin. doi: 10.1109/CBMS.2005.24.

41. A. Nayyar, D. N. Le, & N. G. Nguyen (Eds.). (2018). Anand Nayyar, Dac-Nhuong Le, Nhu Gia Nguyen, Advances in Swarm Intelligence for Optimizing Problems in Computer Science. CRC Press.

42. M. Dorigo (2007). In The Editorial of the First Issue of: Swarm Intelligence Journal. Springer Science + Business Media, LLC, 1(1), 1–2.

43. T. Y. Tan, L. Zhang, S. C. Neoh, & L. Chee Peng (2018). Intelligent Skin Cancer Detection Using Enhanced Particle Swarm Optimization. Knowledge-Based Systems, 158, 118–135, ISSN 0950-7051. doi:10.1016/j.knosys.2018.05.042.

44. M. G. Feshki and O. S. Shijani (2016), "Improving the heart disease diagnosis by evolutionary algorithm of PSO and Feed Forward Neural Network," 2016 Artificial Intelligence and Robotics (IRANOPEN), Qazvin, 2016, pp. 48–53. doi: 10.1109/RIOS.2016.7529489.

Swarm Intelligence and Evolutionary Algorithms for Cancer Diagnosis

Bandana Mahapatra

School of Mechnatronics, Symbiosis Skills and Open University, Pune, India

Anand Nayyar

Graduate School, Duy Tan University, Da Nang, Viet Nam

2.1 INTRODUCTION

Cancer is considered as one of the deadly diseases in medical science, which is characterized by abnormal growth rate of cells in human body. It is described as an outcome of cellular changes that cause uncontrollable frequency of growth which spreads to other body parts if left untreated. Certain cancer types may cause rapid generation of cells in the form of tumors while others may reduce down the production rate to be overtly slow (e.g. leukemia), making both the conditions as life-threatening [1].

Every cell in the body is associated with a fixed life span, after which it dies naturally, which is termed as *apoptosis*. *Apoptosis* is a process by which a cell receives instruction to die which is thereafter replaced by a newer cell that functions comparatively in a better manner [2].

The cancerous cells are ones that lack the component needed to stop the whole process of cell division and death, making them carry on with their division activity for a prolonged lifetime. These tissues and cells accumulated in the body take the form of body outgrowths referred to as lumps that absorb the nutrients and oxygen, which are meant for other cells [3]. The cancerous cells can form tumors, destroy the immune system, and may cause changes that prevent the body from functioning normally [4].

There are numerous methods of treating cancer, such as chemotherapy, immunotherapy, radiation therapy, stem-cell transmission, and surgery. Apart from these, there are other disease-specific treatments that may be adopted with other therapies in combination, in order to maximize the effect over the cancer cells. The doctors usually prescribe the treatment depending on the stage of the cancer along with person's overall health [5].

The cancer cells begin at one part, spread out to other parts with time, affecting the whole body gradually, via *lymph nodes* i.e. the cluster of immunization cells located all over the body. The spreading of cancer cells to other parts is medically termed as *metastasis*, which can be prevented by early treatment, making the need of early cancer detection all the more vital as a contribution to improve the cancer survival rate all over the world [6].

The occurrence of cancer in human body diagnosed at an early nascent stage has more chances of successful treatment when compared to later or advanced stages where spreading of these malign cells makes the treatment all the more difficult reducing the survival chances [7,8]. The cancer survival rate of patients are the maximum at Stage IA being 71%, which slowly reduces to 57% at Stage IB, and consequently lowers down to 46%, 33%, 20%, 14%, 9% and 4% during Stages IIA, IIB, IIIA, IIIB, IIIC and IV at both early and later stage of cancer detection over a period of 5 years as reported by *National Cancer Institute's SEER Databases*.

The above study motivated many researchers to propose as well as formulate various techniques and algorithms that can help the medical professionals for early diagnosis of cancer in a human body, which could contribute in decreasing the death rates [9,10].

The chapter discusses different facets of cancer detection, followed by various *swarm intelligence* as well as *evolutionary algorithms* (EA) that support or claim to facilitate an early detection of cancer of various kinds. Section 2.2 focuses over the biological origin of cancer, various classes the cancers are segregated into, its stages, and its detection modes. Section 2.3 highlights the challenges faced by medico practitioners while detecting cancer cells existing in the body. Section 2.4 discusses about applying various swarm intelligence approaches with an aim to identify occurrences of cancer in the human body. Section 2.5

highlights EA proposed for cancer detection, and finally the chapter is concluded in Section 2.6.

2.2 CLASSIFICATION OF CANCER

The classification of cancer is an important requirement that helps in identification of an appropriate treatment which would help determining the prognosis. The development of cancer cells occurs in progressive manner at an exponential rate after there is occurrence of alteration in the cells genetic structure. Cancers may be biologically categorized in two ways, i.e. type of tissue in which the cancer originates (histological type), and by primary site, or the location in the body where the cancer first developed. This change results in cells suffering an uncontrolled growth pattern [11,12].

In general, cancer types are often categorized based on the following criteria:

(1) Site of origin of the malignant cells

(2) The histology of cell analysis (grading)

(3) The extent of disease (called staging)

Site of cancer origin: This kind of classification highlights the types of tissues in which the cancer cell begins its development. Few examples of site of origin classification types are:

- **Adeno-carcinoma**: Originating in the glandular tissue.

- **Blastoma**: Originates in the embryonic tissue of organs.

- **Carcinoma**: This originates in the epithelial tissue (i.e. tissues that lines the organs and tubes)

- **Leukemia**: This originates in the tissues forming the blood cells.

- **Lymphoma**: These cancer cells originate in the lymph nodes or extra-nodal lymphoid tissue.

- **Sarcoma**: This originates in the connective and supporting tissues, e.g. bone, cartilage, muscles.

Tumor Grading: The grading is a process of analyzing tumor cells obtained through biopsy under a microscope. The range of abnormality shown by cells specifies the grade of cancer. The grade of cancer increases with the increase in the abnormality found in the cells, i.e. from grade 1 to grade 4, as shown in Figure 2.1. The cells that can be uniquely identified, or are different from others, resemble to huge extent to a matured specialized cell, whereas the undifferentiated ones are excessively abnormal immature as well as primitive [12].

The four-gradation applicable over the cells are:

Grade 1. The cells are slightly abnormal and well differentiated.

Grade 2. Cells are more abnormal as well as moderately differentiated.

Grade 3. Cells are quite abnormal and poorly differentiated.

Grade 4. Cells seems to be immature and undifferentiated.

Cancer Staging: The concept of staging is about mode of classifying the extent of the disease as seen in Figure 2.1, i.e. the effectiveness of the cancer within a body.

The TNM system (tumor, node and metastases) can categorize the cancer with respect to the following parameters [14]:

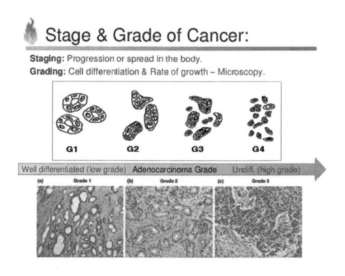

FIGURE 2.1   Stage and Grades of Cancer [13]

- **Tumor size** (T), degree of regional spread or node involvement (N)

- And distant metastasis (M) where,

  Tumor (T) stages are defined as:

  T_0—no evidence of tumor

  T_{1S}—carcinoma is detected in situ (i.e. limited to surface cells)

  T_{1-4}—increasing tumor size and involvement

  Node (N)
  N_0: No Lymph nodes involvement
  N_{1-4}: Increasing degree of lymph nodes involvement
  N_x: The involvement of lymph node is unable to be accessed
  Metastasis (M)
  M_0: No evidence of distant metastasis
  M_1: Evidence of distance metastasis
  A numerical system is also used to classify the extent of disease.

Various stages of cancer are:
  Stage 0: Cancer is restricted to surface cells
  Stage I: Cancer is limited to the tissue of origin, evidence of tumor growth
  Stage II: Cancerous cells spreading is limited to local areas
  Stage III: Extensive local and regional spread
  Stage IV: Distant metastasis observation

Primarily, the international standard of classification as well as nomenclature of histology can also be referred to as the international classification of disease of oncology.

With regards to histological standpoint, there is huge variety of cancers which can be grouped into six major categories [14]:

- Carcinoma

- Sarcoma

- Myeloma

- Leukemia

- Lymphoma

- Mixed types

Carcinoma: The carcinoma is a class of cancer that refers to the presence of malignancy at the neoplasm of the epithelial origin or in other words is medically termed as the cancer of the internal or external lining of the body. This kind of malignancy is seen in almost 80–90% of cancer cases. The presence of epithelial tissue can be found throughout the human body, which includes skin, lining of organs, internal passage ways such as gastro intestinal tract etc. The carcinoma types may be segregated into two broad subcategories:

(1) Adenocarcinoma: area of development is gland or organ.

(2) Squamous cell carcinoma: area of development is squamous epithelium.

The adenocarcinoma cancer type is often found occurring in the mucus membrane. They first appear as a thickened plaque like white mucosa. They are often found to be expanding through the soft tissues where they occur appearing in many areas of body.

Most of the carcinoma types affect the organs or glands where secretion occurs, e.g. breast, lungs, colon, prostrate, bladder etc.

Sarcoma: Sarcoma is a cancer type which can be seen occurring in supportive and connective tissues, e.g. bones, tendons, cartilage, muscles or fats, often affecting young adults. The most common form of sarcoma develops as a painful mass over the bone. The sarcoma tumors usually resemble the tissues where they grow [15], e.g. osteosarcoma or osteogenic sarcoma (bone).

- Chondro sarcoma (cartilage)

- Leiomyo sarcoma (smooth muscles)

- Rhabdomyo sarcoma (skeletal muscles)

- Mesothelial Sarcoma or Mesothelioma (membranous living of body cavities)

- Fibro Sarcoma (fibrous tissues) [16].

Myeloma: The myeloma is a kind of cancer that can be seen originating in the plasma cells of the bone marrow. The plasma cells produce a kind of protein which can be found in the blood.

Leukemia: The leukemia or "liquid cancers" are the cancers of bone marrows which cause an overproduction of white blood cells in the patient's body. The white blood cells produced in the body are immature in nature failing to protect the body from infections. Hence the patients suffering from leukemia are often prone to infections. The leukemia also affects the RBC in the blood resulting in poor blood clotting as well as tiredness due to anemia.

(1) Myelogenous or granulocytic leukemia malignancy found in myloid and granulocytic WBC series.

(2) Lymphatic/lymphocytic or lymphoblastic leukemia: Here abnormality can be seen in lymphoid, lymphocytic blood cell series.

(3) Polycythemia vera or erythremia (here the abnormality of the varying blood cells products while the RBCs are predominant [17,18].

Lymphoma: The lymphoma occurs in glands or nodes of the lymphatic system, network of vessels, nodes, and organs (like spleen, tonsil, thymus etc.), which contributes in purification of body fluids resulting in production of white blood cells or lymphocytes. The lymphomatic cancers are also termed as solid cancers. The lymphomas may even occur in specific organs like stomach, breast, brain; these lymphomas are even referred to as extraordinary lymphomas.

The lymphomas may further be classified into two subcategories based on the presence of Reed Stenberg Cells, which is medically termed as "*Hodgekin Lymphoma*," whereas the other kind is "*non-hodgekin*" lymphoma where the classified cells are absent.

Mixed types—The mixed types are the cancerous tissues that may belong to one or many categories:

- Adenosquamous carcinoma

- Mixed misodermal tumor

- Carcino sarcoma

- Terato carcinoma

The tumor type can be categorized into

(1) Malignant tumors

(2) Benign tumors

Malignant tumors: These tumor types are the cancerous cells that may concur as well as destroy surrounding healthy tissues that include various organs. Here the cancer of the body may spread out to various parts of the body via the blood stream or lymphatic system.

Benign tumors: The benign tumors neither grow at an uncontrollable rate nor either invade neighboring tissues. They generally do not spread out through the body.

There are about more than 200 different varieties of known cancers effecting the human population, majority of them being named after the organs where they occur [19].

2.3 CHALLENGES IN CANCER DIAGNOSIS

For a majority of human diseases, it is always desirable to follow the rule "Prevention is better than cure," where contribution is toward improving the chances of increase in the success rate as well as adopting cost-effective mode of treating the patients. In cancer early diagnosis and the process of non-evasive imaging like CT, MRI, and PET scans often termed as "radiomics" have proven to be increasingly effective in differentiating indolent from aggressive tumors [20,21].

2.3.1 Methods of Cancer Detection

The development of cancer cells or tissues can generally be identified by appearance of signs, symptoms, via screening process.

Screening—the process of screening supports in early detection of cancer cells before visibility or appearance of related symptoms. It is always easy to treat an abnormal tissue or cancer at an early stage since by the time symptoms appear the cancer is probably grown spreading out across, making the treatment all the more harder as well as incurable; on the other hand, a doctor suggesting the screening test does not always indicate it is a cancer. People who are suspected suffering from cancer are investigated with medical tests which include blood tests, X-rays, MRIs, biopsy, pap smear, CT scan, endoscopy and much more.

The biopsy test performed over an infected tissue provides the basic information such as its histological grade, genetic abnormalities and other features. Together this information is useful to evaluate the prognosis and choosing the best treatment available. Apart from these tests, cytogenetics and immunohistochemistry are other kinds of tissue tests. These tests provide information about molecular changes, such as mutations, fusion genes and numerical chromosome changes, which may also indicate the prognosis and best treatment [22,23].

2.3.2 Issues and Challenges Faced While Cancer Detection Process

- In order to aid the process of surgery and guide the surgeons, improved imaging technology contributes in defining as well as removing the tumor margins,while the image recognition software can now classify the melanomas [24]. However, these interventions are expensive which also increase an individual exposure to radiation and have false positive rates.

- The glucose analog F-flude-oxyglucose component used for PET imaging is used to measure the glycolytic flux of cancer cells based on their characteristics increased glucose uptake. This in conjugation with the other traces supports the detection of metabolic changes before the occurrence of alteration at the tissue level [25]. Further opportunity taken would help to avail as well as exploit these resources in order to uplift the use of the biomarkers while analyzing patient's therapeutic targets.

- The study on clonal dynamics of tumor initiation using the technologies like data analytics and exome sequencing may help in early detection of presence of cancer. Stressing over anti-cancer approach, like arranging field of immunotherapies, may prove to be promising during the nascent or early stages of the disease quite ahead of patients' immune system being battered by advanced diseases as well as by prior therapeutics.

- Last but not the least, financial constraints also do contribute in creating obstacles for early detection of cancer.

The future aspects of cancer research and development aim at improving the technologies in order to facilitate the early detection of cancer.

The research and collaboration are currently focusing on development of more sophisticated therapeutic, diagnostic and prognostic tools. The complex problems of cancer cells for high order of expertise ranging from basic level research work to disease prevention.

The cancer field is required for promotion of increased open access into resources such as gene expression, radionics data and patients' tissue samples.

It is important to focus over the aspects of rapid improvements in fields of research and technology. Few model examples are culture models and patient-derived Xenograft Models, and many more novel approaches are built which could work on cultured tumors/models or various other comprehensive analysis in future. The mode of standardizing cry observations includes tissue to be rusticated; studies aiming at improving the process of cancer pathology may move all the way from structural analysis to functional studies offering a positive approach toward patients and R&D.

2.4 APPLYING SWARM INTELLIGENCE ALGORITHM FOR CANCER DIAGNOSIS

Swarm intelligence is a concept built upon the cumulative behavior fragmented, self-organized individual system though natural or artificial. The idea is generally incorporated on "artificial intelligence," the term conceptualized in year 1989 by Wang and Beni [26] with the context to cellular robotics system. The SI-based technology has a varied range of contributions in form of application designed as well as implemented to solve various real-life problems. Recently, the SI approach has been explored to solve various problems related to medical fields such as disease diagnosis, prediction treatment screening, etc.

Few typical SI algorithms exploited in the field of mechanical science are particle swarm optimization (PSO), ACO, Artificial Immune Recognition System (AIRS), artificial weed bee, evasive weed optimization, etc. Majority of these approaches aim at extracting an optimal solution especially in problem areas that are hard to solve. They initiated with the base-level population of agents that simultaneously grow and distribute over with the problem space. Every agent of the population depends on the cooperation and competitive theory that began to explore and exploit. The exploration and exploitation process are done iteratively at a finite step [27].

This section explores the various SI algorithms proposed as well as conceived and conceptualized for early detection of various kinds of cancer till date considered for treatment occurring in the human body.

2.4.1 SI Algorithms for Detection of Lung Cancer

As such, any cancer occurring in the body is deadly, so is lung cancer. Lung cancer is said to be a major cause of death due to cancer worldwide. Early detection of lung cancer is a challenging task due to the structure of cancer cells where the majority of cells are overlapping in nature. Researchers have tried to propose various methodologies with an aim to aid early detection of cancer cells in human body. The technology provided by best et al. [28] is primarily based on PSO-enhanced algorithm which helps in selection of efficient RNA biomarkers, panels, and platelets from RNA sequencing libraries ($n = 779$). The blood-based biopsy for detecting the presence of cancer generally consists of tumor-educated blood platelets (TEPs), which emerge as promised biomarker sources for non-evasive detection of cancer. They have proposed an NSCLC diagnostics classification algorithm based upon the differentially spliced platelet RNAs which use the matched NSCLC/non-cancer platelets cohorts. They have begun with the enhancement of data robustness of data normalization procedure of previously developed SVM-based Thrombo Sequencing Classification algorithm by introducing the process of removing unwanted variation (RUV)-based iterative correction modules, which on the other hand reduce the relative inter-sample variability ($p < 0.0001$, $n = 263$, Student's t-test). They have also implemented the PSO-driven meta-algorithm for pitching out the genes that have more contribution for the classification process. In general, the PSO-driven algorithm makes use of many candidate solutions where by adopting the swarm intelligence and practical velocity the algorithm repeatedly searches for more number of optimal solutions ultimately reaching out to the most optimal fit.

Using the developed algorithm, the researchers have claimed that PSO-driven thrombo sequence platforms allows the selection of a robust biomarker for a blood-based cancer diagnosis, independent of any bias introduced by factors such as age, smoking habits, blood storage time and certain specific inflammatory disease. Apart from this, Asuntha et al. [29] have also proposed an algorithm developed from PSO using Genetic Optimization and SVM technique for the process of feature selection as well as classification. The enhanced process of filtration is claimed to act as a de-noising factor for segmented medical images.

The same concept has been further used by authors in detection of breast cancer which is discussed next.

2.4.2 Swarm Intelligence for Breast Cancer

Apart from other cancers, one of the most common forms of cancer occurring among women is breast cancer whose accountability of death rate is almost more than 60,000 among 1 million cases occurring world-wide every year. The most effective method of reducing death rate is early detection of cancer, which has motivated many researchers to propose and device various algorithms to facilitate the process of initial diagnosis. Majority algorithmic contribution proposed in this area can be credited to genetic algorithm (GA), but researchers have tried PSO method which has proved itself to be comparatively more effective in specific cases specially while considering optimization as a requirement like PSO meta-heuristic optimization can be used for both improving accuracy of diagnosis as well as to overcome the weakness. Apart from this it can also be used for feature selection as well as optimization purpose.

2.4.3 Swarm Intelligence for Ovarian Cancer

Ovarian cancer is rated as the fifth most common cancer type causing death rate of about 74% in 100,000 women in the United States and it is treated as the fourth most common cancer type worldwide. Considering the gravity of the case and its resulting device rate, researchers have tried to formulate algorithm that could detect the abnormality/occurrence of cancer tissues at an early stage. Such research contribution has been proposed by Yan Meng (New Jersey, USA) [30] where he has used a hybridized version of ACO/PSO Algorithm in order to identify the diagnostic proteomic patterns of biomarkers to identify ovarian cancer at a nascent stage.

2.4.4 SI Algorithm for Early Detection of Gastro Cancer

The ACO-based LDA algorithms have been originally developed for the purpose of spectral feature selection to identify the diagnostically useful Raman features of in vivo gastric tissue—Raman spectra for correlation purpose with the gastric tissue pathologies. The algorithm parameters balanced the exploitation–exploration tradeoffs and were adjusted by trial and error to a high convergence rate in order to obtain the best subset of Raman variables for tissue distinction.

2.4.5 Swarm Intelligence for Treating Nano-Robots

The futuristic view of the medical field as conceived and proposed by Adriano Cavalcanti, (Chairman, CEO of CAN Center for Automation of Nano Biotech NPO) [31] are nano-robots which can be quite useful in various implicational areas in the field of medicine as well as the space technology. The nano-robots are mainly expected to be useful for maintaining as well as protecting the body against the pathogene. The theoretical design of the nanorobots has been undergoing various changes since quite a number of decades, which involves integration of fields like nano-biotechnology that provide wide variety of biological molecules with sensory, motor action, artificial intelligence, etc. [32,33,46].

The nano-robots incorporating the swarm behavior include designing the biological traits like stigmergy, decentralization, bifurcations, positive-negative feedbacks, etc. [47]

The concept of ACO integrated with nano-robotics as proposed by Nada et al. [34] has their main steps of algorithm as

P_T = pheromone trail
Step 1. Set initial parameters
Step 2. Set initial pheromone trails
Step 3. While (Result is not obtained)
        Ant solution is constructed
        Local search applied
        Checking for best tour
        P_T ← best tour updation
Step 4. End

The swarm intelligence approach assigned to a medical nano-robot can prove to be successful in attaining the aim of early diagnosis of cancer site in a human body.

The concept designed is, if a swarm of nano-robots is injected into the human muscular system, they would move randomly with the blood flow leaving the pheromone trail behind. These trails would be beneficial in attracting other nano-robots, whereas one that has drifted far off would eventually be lost moving away without detecting the chemical concentration from target route.

The route with high concentration gradient would undergo update quite frequently by pheromones eventually developing as the only traffic route to target site from the site of origin.

Since the nano-robots launch are highly dependent on the blood flow and it is almost impossible to lay a pheromone trail against flow in the body. The resultant of the above algorithm may lead to collapse of the entire system with the loss of adaptability [35]. Moreover, being a probabilistic approach, ACO may not guarantee complete exploration of all the possible sites, since after obtaining the shortest route, swarms may not explore and cure the other areas that might be cancer infected leading to collision of nano-robots among themselves. Considering these aspects further, PSO was proposed by Eberhart and Kennedy in 1995 [36] inspired from behavior of flocking of birds and schooling of fishes, which claimed to provide a complete control over mobility factor of the nano-robots.

The PSO Algorithm is given as

Step 1. Population is initialized to I_0.
Step 2. While (target ≠ result)
   Calculate particles fitness value
   Best particle in system is modified
   Best particle is selected
   Particle position is updated
Step 3. End of while

Apart from PSO, artificial bee colony is also proposed by Karaboga. in 2005 [37], designed considering the behavioral aspect of bees where the whole approach is conceived with the target to find the best solution of the problem.

The algorithm conceived is given as:

Step 1. Initial Population
Step 2. While (Target ≠ Result)
   The employed bees are placed over food source
   The onlooker bees are placed on food source basing on nectar
   deposited

Send scouts to search area with a target to look for new food
source
Memorize the best food source
Step 3. End while

Thereafter, the chemical-based ABC was proposed where artificial bees concept was combined with the pheromone concept of ACO in order to create definite traffic routes. These traffic routes are claimed to overcome the issue of blocking blood vessels resulting due to swarm movements within the blood [38]. The approach is given by the algorithm:

Step 1. Initializing the population to I_0
Step 2. While (target ≠ achieved)

- Activate target-specific sensor for looking out for activated nano-robots

- Threshold value calculation of target molecules and switching of sensors

- In order to find swarm, attractant specific sensor is activated

- RF signals activates inactive worker nano-robots

- Calculate threshold value for the target molecules, worker nano-robots deliver drugs

Step 3. End while.

In year 2014, Kung-Jeng Wang and Kun-Huang Chen [39] proposed a PSO-based algorithm that is capable of collecting the appropriate genes from the gene pool that could identify the cancer. The methodology proposed used decision tree as the classifier. The methodology of using PSO for appropriate gene selection was previously proposed by many researchers like García-Nieto et al. [40], who proposed a modified PSO for high dimensional micro array data augmenting SVM and GA and performing a comparison over six public cancer data sets. Later on, Li et al. used the same technique combining PSO with GA and adapting SVM as the classifier for the gene selection. Thereafter, Mohammad et al. [41] presented an improvised binary PSO in combination with SVM classifier to select near optimal subset of informative gene relevant to cancer classification. Recently, in year 2018, a Novel Hybrid Framework (NFH) was presented which is capable of collecting genes as well as classifying cancer for a high dimensional micro-array data by combining the information gain, F-score, GA, PSO and SVM as presented next.

Apart from the research & development, even companies like Google have conceived various AI tools that can identify the tumors mutation from an image [42]. Scientist have trained an off-the-shelf Google Deep Algorithm which can efficiently differentiate the occurrences of tumor for two common types of lung cancers with an accuracy level of 97%. Similar kind of tool for cancer detection by merely looking at the pathology reports were developed built upon the machine learning techniques [43,44].

2.5 APPLYING EVOLUTIONARY ALGORITHM FOR CANCER DETECTION

The EA concept has also been derived from nature. Since the inception of GA proposed by John Holland in year 1975, EA has also undergone exploration by various researchers, leading to its emergence as a popular research field [45]. Since last two decades, various applications have been successfully proposed in the past 20 years.

The EA concept begins with randomly initialized group of population evolving across several generations. The fittest gene individuals are thereafter selected as parent for the next generation. These genes perform crossover in order to generate new offspring individuals. The randomly selected groups of off-springs are then chosen to undergo mutation followed by selection conducted by algorithm for optimal individuals for survival to the next generation according to survival selection scheme designed beforehand.

The pseudo code of a typical EA is given in algorithm:

Step 1. Initialize variables i = 0
Step 2. Initialize Population [p(i)]
Step 3. Evaluate p(i)
Step 4. While (stop condition ≠ true)
        p(i) ← variation [p(i)]
        Evaluate p(i);
        p(i+1)= select [p(i)]
        i=i+1
Step 5. End while

Few typical examples of EAs are:

- Genetic Algorithm

- Genetic Programming

- Evolutionary Strategy

Among the various classical algorithms, GAs have been adopted widely by the researchers who are formulating concepts for early diagnosis of various forms of cancer in human body.

This section explores the various forms of cancer in human body . The section explores the various strategies, formulated or algorithms proposed by the researchers claiming to aid early detection of cancer among suffering patients at an early stage.

Genetic Algorithm: GA, as described, is one of the most classic EA based on Darwin's Evolution Theory. It is almost hard to distinguish between a GA and an EA.

A typical GA may be explained as a group of initial population where each individual has a fixed-length binary array as its genotype. The fitness of each individual can be divided by the average fitness to calculate the normalized probability to be selected. The algorithm thereafter adopts this approach to select parents for single-point cross-over in order to produce offspring. A typical pseudocode for GA can be given as [48]:

Step 1. Initialize variables i=0;
Step 2. Initialize_Population [p(i)] ← 0; {Initializing the population}
Step 3. Evaluation_Population ← evaluate [P(i)]; {evaluation of population}
Step 4. While (Termination Condition ≠ Satisfied)
  p′(i) ← Variation [p(i)]; {Create new solution}
  Evaluation_population [p′(t)]; {Evaluates the new solutions}
  P(i+1)← Apply Genetic Operation [p′(i) Ù Q]; {population of the next generation}
  i=i+1
Step 5. End while

Basing on this concept, various researchers have tried formulating hybrid improvised algorithm that could prove advantageous in detecting presence of various algorithms. Such kind of research work was taken up in year 2004 by Houlihan et al. [49], where he utilized GA concept as a mode of feature selection for the SVM and artificial neural network which could classify the status of lung cancer among suffering patients. They have claimed that GA can successfully identify the genes that classify the stage and status of a lung cancer with notable predictive performance. In year 2017, Odeh et al. [50] have proposed improvised GA for determining stage of the Lung Cancer to the highest level of accuracy.

Similar methods were adopted for breast cancer prediction where an Ensemble method based on GA was proposed by Chauhan and Swami in year 2018 [51]. They performed a comparative analysis of GA, PSO and differential evolution in their article where the resultant shows GA outperforming the others for weighted average methods. They also conducted an experiment to compare GA-based weighted average method and classical ensemble method where the result shows GA-based weighted average method outperforming the classical ensemble method.

Zhou et al. [52] proposed a framework designed upon neural network and GA as a means to improve the doctor's experience for the diagnosis of illness. Similar contribution has been made by Lambrou, et al. in year 2010 [53], proposed a conformal predictor (CP), the kind of machine learning algorithm that makes use of the evolved rule sets generated by a GA where the rule-based GA has an advantage of being human readable. They applied the methodology over two data set type for testing, i.e. breast cancer as well as ovarian cancer which showed the accuracy level same as that of a classical along with reliability and confidentiality as a measure.

Similar experimental analysis has been done in year 2014 by Rigel et al. [54] who claim that GA-based approach gives better results when prediction accuracy is the objective.

Genetic Programming: While considering the AI concept, GP is a technique where the computer programs are encoded as a set of genes which can be modified via EAs. One of the fundamental problems in computer science is to get the computer work without giving it a proper set of instruction regarding how to do. This challenge is addressed by GP which provides a method for automatically creating work computer program from a high-level problem statement. The working principle of GP is genetically breeding a population of computer programs based on principle of Darwinian's theory of natural selection and biologically inspired operations which includes, reproduction, crossover, mutation and architecture altering operations patterned after gene application and the gene deletion in nature.

The GP may be defined as a domain-independent method which genetically breeds the computer programs in order to solve a problem. The technique of GP iteratively converts a population of computer programs into a novel program generation by applying analogues of naturally occurring genetic operations which includes the process like crossover, mutation, reproduction, gene duplication and gene deletion.

The execution steps of the genetic programming can be given as:

Step 1. Random creation of Initial Population

Step 2. While (Termination criteria ≠ true)

- Execute (Program ∈ population)

- Select one/two individual programs from the population with the probability based on fitness measure

- Create (new individual program), for the population by applying the genetic operations with specified probabilities.

  (a) Reproduction: Copy (Selected Individual Program → new population)

  (b) Crossover: Create (new offspring) for new population by recombining randomly chosen parts from two selected programs

  (c) Mutation: Create one new offspring program for new population by randomly mutating a randomly chosen part of a randomly selected program

  (d) Architecture: Altering operations; choosing an architecture altering operations from the available pool of such operations and create a single offspring program for the new population by applying the chosen architecture altering operation to one selected program.

Step 3. Termination: the criteria ones satisfied, the single best program produced during the run belonging to the population produced during the run. If run is successful, the result may be accurate solution to the problem.

Using this concept of EAs, easy and fast detection of melanoma in human body was enhanced by Rigel et al. [55], who proposed a combination of computer vision techniques along with knowledge of dermatology in order to evolve better technique for the solution. According to the article, the process of image classifications can significantly contribute in diagnosis of disease by the process of accurately identifying the morphological structure of the skin lesions that are responsible for development of cancer cells. They claim that the emerging field of GP carries the potential to evolve better solutions for the process of image classification problems in comparison to other existing methods.

Similar enhanced framework has been proposed by Ryan et al. in [56], in which they have built stage 1 computer-aided detector for breast cancer using GP. The detector mainly examines the mammogram highlighting the suspicious areas that requires further investigation. The over-conservative approach degenerates marking every mammogram or segment as suspicious, even though missing any suspicious area can be disastrous.

Considering the potential of GP in various fields, Mei Sze Tan, Jing Wei Tan et al. further tried the concept to analyze the oral cancer data sets carrying 31 cases collected from Malaysia Oral Cancer Database and Tissue Bank System (MOCDTBS). Here the feature subsets were automatically selected through GP and the resulting influence were recorded. In addition to this, a comparative analysis was carried out by them between GP performance, SVM and logistic regression where GP outperformed the other two approaches proving itself to be most suitable one.

Evolutionary strategy: Apart from GA and GP, evolutionary strategy is also a methodology which was found to be suitable as well as beneficial for being adopted while designing framework in order to detect occurrence of cancer in human beings. The evolutionary strategy is basically an optimization technique which is based on ideas of evolution. This perspective typically belongs to the general class of evolutionary computation or artificial evolution methods.

The objective of this approach is to maximize the suitability of a collection of candidate solution in the context of an objective function from a domain. The objective here is typically obtained by adoption of dynamic variation as surrogate for *descent with modification* where the amount of modification is adopted dynamically with performance-based heuristics. The remaining contemporary approaches co-adapt the parameters that control the amount of bias in variations among the other candidate solution.

The evolutionary strategy procedure is given by the algorithm which includes the process of truncation selection and mutation:

Step 1. Initialize Variables $\mu=0$, $\lambda =0$
Step 2. $\mu \leftarrow$ Number of parents selected
Step 3. $\lambda \leftarrow$ Number of off springs generated by parents
Step 4. $P \leftarrow \{ \}$ // Initialize the array
Step 5. For ($\lambda \neq$ False)   // Build Initial population
    $P \leftarrow P \cup$ {new random individual}
Step 6. Best $\leftarrow \square$
Step 7. While (Best $\neq$ Ideal Solution || Time $\neq$ Null)
Step 8.   For each $P_i \in P$
     Access_Fitness (P_i)
     If (Best $= \square$ or Fitness (P_i) > Fitness (Best))
      Best $\leftarrow P_i$
     $Q \leftarrow$ the μ individuals in P whose fitness () are greatest//
     Truncation selection
     $P \leftarrow \{\}$
     For (each individual $Q_i \in Q$)
      For (λ/μ)
       P U {Mutate copy (Q_i)}
Step 9. End While

Based on the EA strategies, various researchers have proposed techniques and algorithms that can detect various kinds of cancers.

Belciug et al. [57] have proposed an EA-based strategy for building a framework that could take the decision whether cancer exists or not. They experimented with five kinds of medical data sets consisting of breast cancer and liver fibrosis. Based on the resultant data, the researchers claimed that the proposed model can be adapted easily to different medical decision-making issues and similar decision-making models. They also later on performed a comparative analysis of the proposed framework along with other machine learning techniques.

Apart from generalized cancer detection models, evolutionary strategy was used in designing approaches for the treatment of tumor evolution as a therapeutic target within the evolutionary framework.

Cancer through the perspective of physical science may be treated as a complicated adaptive system that can be appropriately studied in the context of evolution as well as the evolutionary theory. Various tools derived from evolution and evolutionary theory can be experimented for the complex heterogeneous nature of the cancer within a tissue ecosystem, e.g. game theory.

2.6 CONCLUSION

Cancer detection is a vital aspect in the field of medical science because cancer-related death rates are still alarmingly high. It's a threat to human life; forthcoming generations need appropriate means to diagnose, treat and manage different types of cancer or related diseases. With technology advancement and growth in digitalization all over the world, cancer research sectors have also incorporated technological modes for early detection as well as treatment. It is very important to undergo early diagnosis and apt treatment in order to decrease the rate of mortality caused due to cancer.

This chapter provides us with an overview of various kinds of cancers, its classification that includes its various types, stages, and challenges faced during diagnosis. The chapter also covers the methodology regarding the recent tools and technologies used so far in the process of cancer diagnosis. Its major highlights are the various swarm intelligence and EA approaches proposed by various researchers, belonging to industry as well as academia for early detection of cancer among human beings, including the aspects that need to be considered for future research work to be undertaken by scientists.

ACKNOWLEDGEMENT

The authors thank Dr. Shashidhar Venkatesh Murthy, Associate Professor and Head of Pathology in the School of Medicine at James Cook University, Australia, for permission to use Figure 2.1 titled "stages and grade of cancer" in this chapter.

REFERENCES

1. Cancer – Signs and symptoms. NHS Choices. Available at : https://www.nhs.uk/conditions/cancer/symptoms/ (Retrieved 10 March 2019).
2. Cancer. World Health Organization (12 September 2018). Available at: https://www.who.int/health-topics/cancer (Retrieved 19 March 2019).
3. Anand, P., Kunnumakara, A. B., Sundaram, C., Harikumar, K. B., Tharakan, S. T., Lai, O. S.& Aggarwal, B. B. (2008). Cancer is a preventable

disease that requires major lifestyle changes. *Pharmaceutical Research*, 25(9), 2097–2116.

4. National Cancer Institute. (26 February 2018). Targeted Cancer Therapies. Available Online ay: https://www.cancer.gov/about-cancer/treatment/types/ targeted-therapies/targeted-therapies-fact-sheet (Retrieved 28 March 2019).

5. SEER Stat Fact Sheets: All Cancer Sites. (26 September, 2016). National Cancer Institute. Available Online at: https://seer.cancer.gov/statfacts/ (Retrieved 18 March 2019).

6. Vos, T., Allen, C., Arora, M., Barber, R. M., Bhutta, Z. A., Brown, A. & Coggeshall, M. (2016). Global, regional, and national incidence, prevalence, and years lived with disability for 310 diseases and injuries, 1990–2015: a systematic analysis for the Global Burden of Disease Study 2015. *The Lancet*, *388*(10053), 1545–1602.

7. Ro, T. H., Mathew, M. A., & Misra, S. (2015). Value of screening endoscopy in evaluation of esophageal, gastric and colon cancers. *World Journal of Gastroenterology: WJG*, *21*(33), 9693.

8. Defining Cancer. (17 September 2007). National cancer institute. (Retrieved 28 March 2019).

9. Obesity and Cancer Risk. National Cancer Institute. (3 January 2012). (Retrieved 4 April 2019).

10. Jayasekara, H., MacInnis, R. J., Room, R., & English, D. R. (2015). Long-term alcohol consumption and breast, upper aero-digestive tract and colorectal cancer risk: A systematic review and meta-analysis. *Alcohol and Alcoholism*, 51(3), 315–330.

11. World Cancer Report. (2014). World health organization. Chapter 1.1. ISBN 978-92-832-0429-9. (Retrieved 1 April 2019).

12. Cancer classification. (2000). https://training.seer.cancer.gov/disease/ categories/classification.html. (Retrieved 18 May 2019).

13. Pathology of Neoplasia. (2014). www.slideshare.net/vmshashi/pathology-lecture-neoplasia. (Retrieved 18 May 2019).

14. How cancer is diagnosed. (9 March 2015). (Retrieved from www.cancer. gov/about-cancer/diagnosis-staging/diagnosis).

15. Signs and symptoms of cancer. (11 August 2014). (Retrieved from www. cancer.org/cancer/cancer-basics/signs-and-symptoms-of-cancer.html).

16. Symptoms of cancer. (29 March 2018). (Retrieved from www.cancer.gov/ about-cancer/diagnosis-staging/symptoms).

17. Understanding cancer prognosis. (29 August 2018). (Retrieved from www. cancer.gov/about-cancer/diagnosis-staging/prognosis).

18. Ferlay, J., Shin, H. R., Bray, F., Forman, D., Mathers, C., & Parkin, D. M. (2010). Estimates of worldwide burden of cancer in 2008: GLOBOCAN 2008. *International Journal of Cancer*, 127(12), 2893–2917.

19. Van Raamsdonk, C. D., Bezrookove, V., Green, G., Bauer, J., Gaugler, L., O'brien, J. M., … & Bastian, B. C. (2009). Frequent somatic mutations of GNAQ in uveal melanoma and blue naevi. *Nature*, 457(7229), 599.

20. Cerroni, L., Barnhill, R., Elder, D., Gottlieb, G., Heenan, P., Kutzner, H., ... & Kerl, H. (2010). Melanocytic tumors of uncertain malignant potential: Results of a tutorial held at the XXIX Symposium of the International Society of Dermatopathology in Graz, October 2008. *The American Journal of Surgical Pathology*, 34(3), 314–326.

21. Stelow, E. B., Shaco-Levy, R., Bao, F., Garcia, J., & Klimstra, D. S. (2010). Pancreatic acinar cell carcinomas with prominent ductal differentiation: Mixed acinar ductal carcinoma and mixed acinar endocrine ductal carcinoma. *The American Journal of Surgical Pathology*, 34(4), 510–518.

22. Golub, T., Slonim, D., Tamayo, P. et al. (1999). Molecular classification of cancer: Class discovery and class prediction by gene expression monitoring. *Science*, 286(5439), 531–537.

23. Segal, E., Friedman, N., Kaminski, N., Regev, A., & Koller, D. (2005). From signatures to models: understanding cancer using microarrays. *Nature genetics*, 37(6s), S38–345.

24. Esteva, A., Brett Kuprel, R. A., Novoa, J. K., Swetter, S. M., Blau, H. M., & Sebastian, T. (25 February 2017). Dermatologist-level classification of skin cancer with deep neural networks. *Nature*, 542, 115–118.

25. Challapalli, A., & Aboagye, E. O. (2016). Positron emission tomography imaging of tumor cell metabolism and application to therapy response monitoring. *Frontiers in oncology*, 6, 44., US National Library of Medicine-National Institutes of Health, 2016 Feb 29 .

26. Beni, G., & Wang, J. (1993). Swarm intelligence in cellular robotic systems. In *Robots and biological systems: towards a new bionics* (pp. 703–712). Springer, Berlin, Heidelberg.

27. Lones, M. A. (2014, July). Metaheuristics innature-inspired algorithms . In *Proceedings of the Companion Publication of the 2014 Annual Conference on Genetic and Evolutionary Computation* (pp. 1419–14191422). ACM.

28. Best, M. G., GJG, Sjors., Sol, N., & Wurdinger, T. (2019). RNA sequencing and swarm intelligence–enhanced classification algorithm development for blood-based disease diagnostics using spliced blood platelet RNA. *Nature protocols*, 14(4), 1206–1234.

29. Asuntha, A., Singh, N., & Srinivasan, A. (2016). PSO, genetic optimization and SVM algorithm used for lung cancer detection. *Journal of Chemical and Pharmaceutical Research*, 8(6), 351–359. doi:10.1038/s41596-019-0139-5.

30. Meng, Y. (2007). A swarm intelligence based algorithm for proteomic pattern detection of ovarian cancer. 10.1109/CIBCB.2006.331010.

31. Cavalcanti, A. *CEO Chairman, Research Scientist, Inventor, Nanorobot Invention and Linux: The Open Technology Factor.*Article retrieved at https://www.nanotech-now.com/news.cgi?story_id=35023

32. Nayyar, A., & Singh, R. (2017). Ant colony optimization (ACO) based routing protocols for wireless sensor networks (WSN): A survey. *International Journal of Advanced Computer Science and Applications*, 8, 148–155.

33. Nayyar, A., & Singh, R. (2014). A comprehensive review of ant colony optimization (ACO) based energy-efficient routing protocols for wireless sensor networks. *International Journal of Wireless Networks and Broadband Technologies (IJWNBT)*, 3(3), 33–55.
34. Nada, M. A., & Salami, A. (2009). Ant colony optimization algorithm. *UbiCC Journal*, 4(3).824-826
35. Kaewkamnerdpong B., Bentley P.J. (2009) Modelling Nanorobot Control Using Swarm Intelligence: A Pilot Study. In: Lim C.P., Jain L.C., Dehuri S. (eds) Innovations in Swarm Intelligence. Studies in Computational Intelligence, vol 248. Springer, Berlin, Heidelberg
36. Eberhart, R., & Kennedy, J. (1995, November). Particle swarm optimization. In *Proceedings of the IEEE international conference on neural networks* (Vol. 4, pp. 1942-1948).
37. Karaboga, D. (2005). *An idea based on honey bee swarm for numerical optimization* (Vol. 200, pp. 1–10). Technical report-tr06, Erciyes university, engineering faculty, computer engineering department.
38. Sharma, V., & Srivastava, S. (2014). Chemical sensing based ABC Swarm intelligence algorithm for cancer treating nanorobots. *INROADS- An International Journal of Jaipur National University*, 3(1), 101–105.
39. Kung-JengWang, B., & Kun-HuangChen, K.-M. (2014). A hybrid classifier combining SMOTE with PSO to estimate 5-year survivability of breast cancer patients. *Applied Soft Computing*, 20, 15–24.
40. García-Nieto, J., Alba, E., Jourdan, L., & Talbi, E. (2009). Sensitivity and specificity based multiobjective approach for feature selection: Application to cancer diagnosis. Information Processing Letters, 109(16), 887-896. doi:10.1016/j.ipl.2009.03.029.
41. Mohamad, M. S., Omatu, S., Deris, S., Yoshioka, M., Abdullah, A., & Ibrahim, Z. (2013). An enhancement of binary particle swarm optimization for gene selection in classifying cancer classes. *Algorithms for Molecular Biology*, 8(1), 15. .Hindawi Publishing Corporation Computational and Mathematical Methods in Medicine Volume 2012, Article ID 320698, 7 pages doi:10.1155/2012/320698
42. Agravat, R. R., & Raval, M. S. (2018). Deep learning for automated brain tumor segmentation in MRI images. In *Soft Computing Based Medical Image Analysis* (pp. 183–201). Academic Press.Biomedical Image Analysis Group, Imperial College London, UK 2 Microsoft Research, Cambridge, UK
43. Nayyar, A., Puri, V., & Suseendran, G. (2019). Artificial bee colony optimization—population-based meta-heuristic swarm intelligence technique. In V. E. Balas et al. (eds.), *Data Management, Analytics and Innovation* Advances in Intelligent Systems and Computing 839 (pp. 513–525). Springer Nature Singapore Pte Ltd. 2019, Singapore.https://doi.org/10.1007/978-981-13-1274-8_38
44. Durbhaka, G. K., Selvaraj, B., & Nayyar, A. (2019). Firefly swarm: Meta-heuristic swarm intelligence technique for mathematical optimization. In

Data Management, Analytics and Innovation (pp. 457–466). Springer, Singapore.

45. Nayyar, A., & Singh, R. (2016 March). Ant colony optimization—computational swarm intelligence technique. In *2016 3rd International Conference on Computing for Sustainable Global Development* (INDIACom) (pp. 1493–1499). IEEE.

46. Kumar, A., Sangwan, S. R., & Nayyar, A. (2019). Rumour veracity detection on twitter using particle swarm optimized shallow classifiers. *Multimedia Tools and Applications*, 1–19.

47. Nayyar, A., Puri, V., & Le, D. N. (2017). Internet of nano things (IoNT): Next evolutionary step in nanotechnology. *Nanoscience and Nanotechnology*, 7(1), 4–8.

48. Nayyar, A., Garg, S., Gupta, D., & Khanna, A. (2018). Evolutionary computation: Theory and algorithms. In *Advances in Swarm Intelligence for Optimizing Problems in Computer Science* (pp. 1–26). Chapman and Hall/CRC, USA.

49. Houlihan, N. G., Inzeo, D., Joyce, M., Leslie, B.T.. (2004). Symptom Management of Lung Cancer. *Clinical Journal of Oncology Nursing*, 8(6).645-652

50. Odeh, A., Ibrahim, A. A., & Bustanji, A. (2017). Novel Genetic Algorithm for Early Prediction and Detection of Lung Cancer. *Journal of Cancer Treatment and Research*, 5(2), 15–18. doi:10.11648/j.jctr.20170502.1342.

51. Chauhan, P., & Swami, A. (2018 July). Breast cancer prediction using genetic algorithm based ensemble approach. In *2018 9th International Conference on Computing, Communication and Networking Technologies (ICCCNT)* (pp. 1–8). IEEE.Bangalore, India 10.1109/ICCCNT.2018.8493927

52. Zhou, Z. H., Jiang, Y., Yang, Y. B., & Chen, S. F. (2002). Lung cancer cell identification based on artificial neural network ensembles. *Artificial Intelligence Medicine*, 24(1), 25–36.

53. Lambrou, A., Papadopoulos, H., & Gammerman, A. (2010). Reliable confidence measures for medical diagnosis with evolutionary algorithms. *IEEE Transactions on Information Technology in Biomedicine*, 15(1), 93–99.

54. Rigel, D. S., Russak, J., & Friedman, R. (2010). The evolution of melanoma diagnosis: 25 years beyond the ABCDs. *CA: A Cancer Journal for Clinicians*, 60(5), 301–316. doi:10.1186/1742-4682-11-S1-S7.

55. Rigel, D. S., Russak, J., & Friedman, R. (2010). The evolution of melanoma diagnosis: 25 years beyond the ABCDs. *CA: a cancer journal for clinicians*, *60*(5), 301-316. Wiley online library doi:10.3322/caac.20074.

56. Ryan C., Krawiec K., O'Reilly UM., Fitzgerald J., Medernach D. (2014) Building a Stage 1 Computer Aided Detector for Breast Cancer Using Genetic Programming. In: Nicolau M. et al. (eds) Genetic Programming. EuroGP 2014. Lecture Notes in Computer Science, vol 8599. Springer, Berlin, Heidelberg

57. Belciug, S., Gorunescu, F., & Serbanescu, M. (2015). Improving MLP classification accuracy for breast cancer detection through evolutionary computation, partially connectivity and feature selection. *Journal of Biomedical Informatics*, 53, 261–269.

CHAPTER 3

Brain Tumour Diagnosis

Dhananjay Joshi

Department of Computer Engineering, SVKM's NMIMS (Deemed-to-be-University), Mukesh Patel School of Technology Management & Engineering, Shirpur, India

Nitin Choubey

Department of Information Technology, SVKM's NMIMS (Deemed-to-be-University), Mukesh Patel School of Technology Management & Engineering, Shirpur, India

Rajani Kumari

Department of Computer Application and IT, JECRC University, Jaipur, India

3.1 INTRODUCTION

"There exists no machine, science or a technology that can predict 100 percentage accurate future medical diagnosis of any person after next five minutes. To carry out the remedial measures using an experience, skill set and prediction before an incidence happening also has some human limitations. The doctor cannot be always right. Hence, people should neither consider a doctor as a God nor as a criminal."

-Swami Vivekananda

As per above statement, Swami Vivekananda has focused on the core of the medical profession that doctors cannot always make accurate decisions for the diagnosis of any particular disease for a patient since it is also based on accumulated knowledge base through experience, and the knowledge base can never be practically complete and correct. Every knowledge based system always has scope for more and more perfection to make more accurate decisions.

Artificial intelligence (AI) is and can be applied to every field. By combining nature-inspired computing and AI, one can predict the things accurately. In today's world, having advancement in computing technology, it is very easy to solve any problem with the optimal solution, but still many problems exist whose search space is very much large. The problems having large space take more time or are even difficult to track through classical optimization techniques. A diagnosis of a brain tumor is possible using simple model depicted in figure 3.1. It consists of feature extraction and selections, followed by machine learning model for prediction.

Above model accepts brain image as input, and then it works with feature extraction and selections. Feature extraction can be done using edge detection and morphological operations like erosion, dilation or filters. These techniques suffer from various types of image noise. These extracted features will lead to less accurate prediction or diagnosis. If proper features are selected it model will provide accuracy.

If nature-inspired-algorithms (NIA) are used to select features, the model will improve the performance. NIA works very well for any optimization problem [1]. Many complex problems can be solved very easily using NIA. NIA is very popular in the field of optimization and gives the best result [2]. NIA are classified into different classes based on their sources of inspirations [2], i.e., bio inspired algorithms, chemistry inspired and physics inspired algorithm.

This is not the case that above is the final classification of NIAs; one can also classify them in different classes based on some criterion.

Swarm intelligence and evolutionary algorithms are not only intelligent; but also evolutionary techniques for optimization problems. These two are the subclasses of population based optimization algorithm, i.e. swarm intelligence and evolutionary algorithm.

Population-based optimization algorithms can be applied to every field, namely science, engineering, business, healthcare, education, economics, stock predictions, robotics, computer games and various polls like elections, sports tournament predictions, movie awards, etc. Swarm and evolutionary techniques will give a performance guarantee as it is optimized algorithm and gives most suitable solutions. Unanimous AI uses swarm intelligence to predict sporting events, political events, and Oscars too [3,4]. Swarm

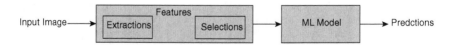

FIGURE 3.1   Simple model for brain tumor diagnosis.

intelligence was also able to predict TIME's Person of the Year for 2017 [5]. Barone and While [6] proposed to use evolutionary algorithms to learn to play games of an imperfect information - in particular, the game of poker. Every disease is a serious disease if it either grows rapidly or reaches to its final stage. Proper, correct and accurate diagnosis of every disease is required to get a cure from it. Heart disease, cancer, and diabetes are some diseases. Cancer is the most common disease. Despite of recent technology and medical progress, cancer is the second leading cause of the death in years 2016 [7], 2017 [8] and 2018 [9].

Cancer is also known as malignancy. Abnormal growth of cells leads to cancer. There are 100+ types of cancers, namely lung, breast, colorectal cancer and prostate are a few of the most common cancers. Brain tumor or cancer is not most common, as brain is an important part of our body without which we cannot function. A brain is the only part which controls all the other organs of the body. Brain tumor and meningitis are diseases of the brain which have serious consequences.

The brain is an important part of our body, and it should function normally and properly, the brain should be free from any disease. Brain tumor diagnosis is very difficult in the initial stage if swelling in the brain is too small or about to start. Brain tumors are of two types: benign and malignant. It can be primary or secondary according to its growth. All brain tumors are not cancerous tumors. Brain tumor scans are MRI and CT.

Lump or swelling which is not having a definite or regular shape is called brain tumor. There are over 130 different brains and spinal tumors, which are grouped according to the type of cell they grow from, their location in the brain, and how rapidly they are likely to grow and spread [10]. The tumor, which is originating in a brain, is known as primary brain tumors. If the tumor started somewhere else in the body, e.g. first lung, then spread to the brain, is known as a secondary brain tumor or metastases.

As per National Brain Tumor Society, In 2018, nearly 700,000 people in the United States had a primary brain tumor, and importantly, more than 86,000 will be diagnosed in the year 2019 [11]. Brain tumors significantly affect quality of life and change everything for a patient and their loved ones. Brain tumor does not discriminate, inflicting men, women, or children of all races and ethnicities. According to National Brain Tumor Society, the average survival rate for all malignant brain tumor patients is only 35%, and an estimated 16,830 people will die from malignant brain tumors (brain cancer) in 2019 [11].

Diagnosis is the process in which cause of the health problem is found. If any patient has a symptom of any disease, after performing some tests, doctor may suggest presence of a particular disease. Diagnosis is the process that may take long time and is frustrating too, but it is important for the healthcare team to rule out other possible reasons for a health problem before making the diagnosis of cancer.

World Health Organization (WHO) classifies the brain tumors in various grades of severity. Severity can be obtained from proper and accurate diagnosis. As per WHO brain tumors are classified as: Astrocytoma, low-grade astrocytoma (grades I and II), high-grade astrocytoma (grades III and IV), ganglioglioma, oligodendroglioma, ependymoma and medulloblastoma. The tumor is more malignant if the grade is higher. Brain tumor grading can help the medical experts to plan treatment and output predictions [12]. Following are the possible tumor grades.

Grade - I: - It is a least malignant tumor; the cells look normal and grow slowly and are usually associated with long-term survival. Surgery is an effective treatment for grade - I. Examples of grade - I are pilocytic astrocytoma, craniopharyngioma, gangliocytoma, and ganglioglioma.

Grade - II: - In this cell looks slightly abnormal and grow slowly.

Grade - III: - Cells look abnormal and actively reproduce abnormal cells in nearby normal brain tissues. Grade - III tends to recur often as a grade IV.

Grade - IV: - Cells look most abnormal and not only very fast growing but also most malignant tumor. Grade IV tumors form new blood vessels so that they can maintain their rapid growth. The example is glioblastoma multiform.

In most of the literature, brain tumors can be diagnosed successfully, but there is presence of noise in the image and accuracy is not good. So NIA can be used to avoid image noise and for improving accuracy. Kumar et al. [13], used exponential spider monkey optimization and SVM for prediction. The model shown in Figure 3.2 is updated and more detailed version of brain tumor image classification.

The model represented in Figure 3.2 consists of three phases- feature extraction, selection, and ML model. Feature extraction is done using image processing strategies. Feature selection is the complex task. NIA have widely been used in many literatures. In our case, pre-processed brain image will be given as input for feature extraction. Image noise and skull removal are the two steps used in pre-processing.

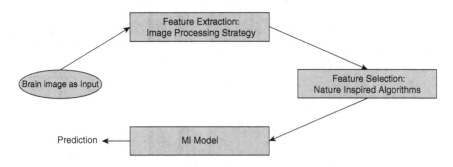

FIGURE 3.2   Brain tumor image classification [13].

Feature Extraction: Conversion of input image into the sets of features is known as feature extraction. Doing brain image analysis and accurate classification one must extract high dimensional features from image. Extracted features can be used for classification of brain tumor. Many feature extraction techniques are available.

Feature Selection: In above phase high-dimensional features are extracted. These features may also contain unwanted features. Such unwanted features

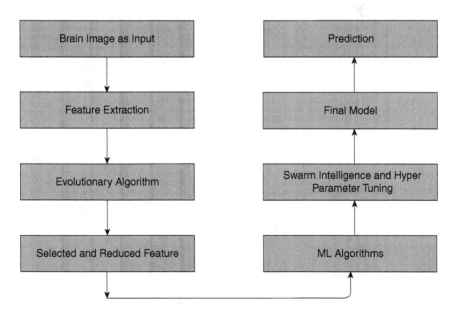

FIGURE 3.3   Applying evolutionary algorithm and swarm intelligence together.

may degrade the performance of the classifier. Feature selection with nature-inspired computing endeavors with an accuracy of the classifier by selecting required features only. A genetic algorithm is the most popular method for feature reduction.

ML Model: The selected features are given as input to classification to classify healthy brain or tumor brain.

One more possible model is represented in Figure 3.3, where evolutionary algorithms for feature selections and swarm intelligence along with the hyper tuning parameters are used to get final model. This model will provide better accuracy as both techniques are working together for more accurate result.

3.2 APPLYING EVOLUTIONARY ALGORITHMS FOR BRAIN TUMOR DIAGNOSIS

3.2.1 Evolutionary Algorithm

Charles Darwin proposed the concept of evolutionary algorithms in 1859. It was inspired by natural selection and evolution. Evolution is continuous process which helps species to adopt the environment changes. We know the world is the dynamic, ever changing in nature and the problems of optimization are too complex. Optimization problems require quick feedback of recent improved solution; it might be success or failure. In evolutionary computational strategies Darwin's principle of survival of fittest is accepted. By adapting Darwin's principle several physical processes are carried out for gaining optimal solution, in short we can say that what selects the best discard the rest. Evolutionary computations are playing major role in designing the models for computer algorithms. This is because in natural world evolution has not only improved life form but also created more complex species through evolution. Basically, evolution is a random process carried out by a simple physical mechanism of mating and mutation. In the mating process, recombination of parents is carried out. Next is a mutation which involves making random changes in produced offspring's.

Nayyar et al. [14] presented evolutionary computation - theory and algorithms, and highlighted the importance of evolutionary algorithms in the real world. Alzubi et al. [15] overviewed machine learning from theory to algorithm in detailed in diversified application areas and discussed about ten categories of machine learning paradigms. Evolutionary learning is one of the paradigm inspired by biological organisms. Evolutionary learning provides best solution and it is based on idea of fitness [15]. Satapathy and Rajinikanth [16] presented JAYA Algorithm (JA) to mine the irregular section of brain MRI, author used JA and Otsu's function for pre-processing state and in post processing, and Chan Vese (CV) to mine irregular section from pre-processed MRI. JA is evolutionary algorithm. Rajasekaran and Gounder [12] discussed about brain tumor segmentation from brain images; in their survey they used three segmentation techniques namely, fuzzy c means, region growing method and evolutionary genetic algorithm.

Evolutionary algorithms are classified as genetic algorithm (GA), genetic programming (GP), evolutionary strategy (ES) and evolutionary programming (EP) and differential evolution (DE).
The characteristics of evolutionary algorithms are [17]:
Flexibility: It can be applied to different types of problems and domains.
Robustness: It can deal with any noise and uncertainty.
Adaptive: It can deal with dynamic environments.
Autonomous: It works without human intervention.
Decentralized: It works without central control.
General steps in evolutionary algorithm are [17]:
Loop: If termination criterion is not satisfied go-to step 1 else go-to end loop

1. Parent solution selection

2. Recombination of pair of parents

3. Mutation of resulting offspring

4. New candidate evaluation solution

5. Selection of the new individuals for the next generation.

End Loop
Figure 3.4 represents general steps followed in evolutionary algorithms. GA, GP, ES, EP and DE are available evolutionary algorithms.

Many of the researchers use GA for brain tumor diagnosis. Vishnulakshmi and Muhamamdu [18] used FCM and GA for detection and segmentation of brain tumor. Kole and Halder [19] used a GA based clustering method for tumor detection and isolation of tumor cells. Sari and Tuna [20] used GA for prediction of pathological subjects. Keerthana and Xavier [21] proposed an intelligent system for early assessment of and

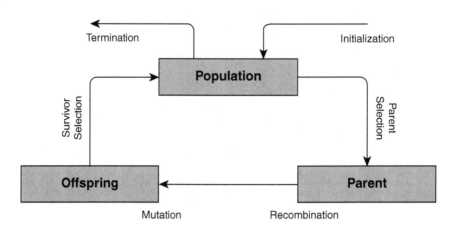

FIGURE 3.4   General steps in evolutionary algorithm [17].

classification of brain tumor using data mining technique and used GA for optimization of features and SVM parameter. A GA and neural network is used by Alalayah et al. [22] for breast cancer diagnosis. GA is used by Johnson et al. [23] for prediction of progression to Alzheimer disease. Rajasekaran and Gounder [12] reviewed papers for brain tumor segmentation.

Genetic Algorithm

It is one of the most important evolutionary algorithms. The main aim is to select best. In case of brain tumor image, high dimensional features will be extracted and GA can be applied to select best and required features.

Pseudo code of Genetic Algorithm
Select high dimensional image feature as population.
Loop: Until stopping criterion is satisfied repeat through
Calculate fitness value for each feature
Selection of the parents
Recombination and mutation
New feature selection for next generation
End loop

3.2.2 Conceptual Framework 1: Applying Evolutionary Algorithm for Brain Tumor Diagnosis.

For this model, pre-processed brain image will be given as input. Feature extraction is the next phase in which high dimensional features are extracted, here any image processing technique can be used. Extracted high dimensional features will be given as input to the evolutionary algorithm to select required features, which provide reduced features and can be further given as input to SVM or CNN as a classifier.

Cross-validation and hyper tuning is done before final model. As per earlier discussion, GA can be used as evolutionary algorithm in Figure 3.5 for diagnosis of brain tumor.

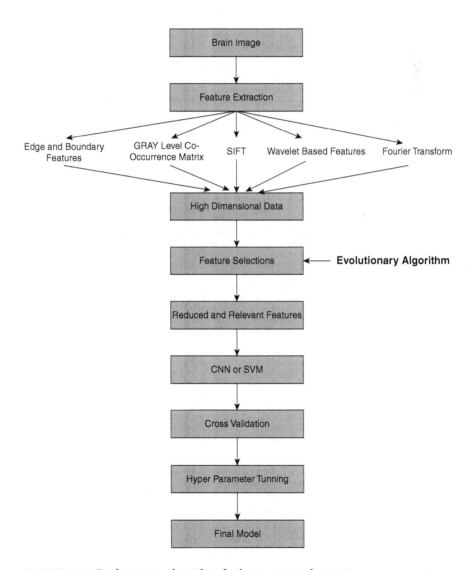

FIGURE 3.5   Evolutionary algorithm for brain tumor diagnosis.

3.3 APPLYING SWARM INTELLIGENCE ALGORITHMS FOR BRAIN TUMOR DIAGNOSIS

3.3.1 Swarm Intelligence (SI) - Based Algorithms

Diagnosis of tumor in the early stage is essential to provide necessary treatment. SI is used in optimization problems, especially in the medical field for the purpose of diagnosis and prediction. Accurate diagnosis is possible using swarm intelligence-based algorithms. Nayyar and Singh [24] defined swarm intelligence as, "any attempt to design algorithm or distributed problem solving devices inspired by the collective behavior of social insects and other animal societies." SI focuses on study of integrated behavior of social insects and other animal socialites. In SI, the individual swarms can interact directly or indirectly [24]. Video or audio mode can be used for direct interaction. Birds interact with each other via specific sound. Bees interact via waggle dance. Indirect interaction is done via environments. Any one swarm agent can change the environment. The example of indirect interaction is ant colony optimization.

G. Beni Hackwood and J. Wang were first to conceptualize swarm intelligence in 1989. Nayyar et al. [25] provided the details about the swarm intelligence based - techniques available till 2018, comprehensively with their mathematical proofs in the book titled "Advances in Swarm Intelligence for Optimizing Problems in Computer Science" [25], includes evolutionary algorithm, GA, swarm intelligence, Ant Colony Optimization (ACO), Particle Swarm Optimization (PSO), Artificial Bee Colony (ABC), Firefly Swarm Optimization, Bat Algorithm, Cuckoo Search Algorithm, Glow-Worm Algorithm, WASP Swarm Optimization, Fish Swarm Optimization, and book also includes many miscellaneous swarm intelligence techniques such as Termite Hill Algorithm, Cockroach Swarm Optimization, the Monkey Search Algorithm, the Bumblebee algorithm, the Social Spider Optimization Algorithm, Cat Swarm Optimization, Intelligent Water Drop, Dolphin Echolocation, Biogeography-Based Optimization, the Paddy Field Algorithm, the Weightless Swarm Algorithm, Eagle Strategy.

Nayyar et al. [26] highlighted swarm intelligence, not only to enable researcher to understand various issues swarm intelligence and swarm robotics but also to clear the foundation of swarm intelligence with various concepts like metaheuristics swarm, technical terms such as collective intelligence, adaptability and diversity. Kamble and Rane [27] represented, brain tumor segmentation from MRI, using ACO. It segmented tumor portion accurately.

Swarm intelligence follows AREAS meaning space or region. AREAS are principles of swarm intelligence namely awareness, resiliency, expandability, autonomy, solidarity. Self-organization and division of labour are the most important necessary properties of swarm intelligence.

3.3.2 Self-Organization:

This is a set of dynamical mechanisms which result in structures at the global level of a system by means of interactions among its low-level components. These mechanisms show the basic rules for the interactions between the components of the system. The rules make sure that the interactions are executed purely by local information without any relation to the global pattern. It is based on following characteristics - [28]

- Positive feedback: - It is information extracted from output of system and given as input to promote convenient structure. It accelerates the system to a new stable state.

- Negative feedback: - Compensate the effect of positive feedback and helps to stabilize the collective pattern.

- Fluctuation: - Are the rate or magnitude of random changes in the system.

- Multiple interaction: - Provides the way of learning from the individuals within the society and thus enhance the combined intelligence of the swarm.

3.3.3 Division of Labor:

It is a cooperative labor in specific, circumscribed tasks and like roles. In a group, there are various tasks, which performed simultaneously by specialized individuals. Simultaneous task performance by cooperating specialized individuals is believed to be more efficient than the sequential task performance by unspecialized individuals.

3.3.4 Particle Swarm Optimization

PSO is developed by Kennedy and Eberhart in 1995[29]. Banchpalliwar and Salankar [30] presented, how Fuzzy C-Means (FCM) and PSO techniques improves the accuracy over FCM. Zamani and Nadimi-Shahraki [31], extracted efficient pattern from breast cancer using PSO then ANN is applied for classification. Their experimental results show PSO gives high accuracy of diagnosis. PSO is used by Punidha et al. [32] for segmentation of brain tumor. Gunavathi and Premalatha [33] discussed about various feature selection techniques, namely PSO and Cucu Search in cancer classification. Adithyan et al.[34] discussed about PSO and firefly. Muslim et al. [35] used PSO for breast cancer diagnosis. As PSO is one of the modern heuristic algorithms based on swarm intelligence, which makes the segmentation process more efficient compared to GA and ACO [36]. Comparative study of PSO and ACO by Selvi and Umarani [37] concludes that the PCO is better than ACO. Durbhaka et al. [38] reviewed firefly algorithm. Nayyar et al. [39] presented artificial bee colony in a detailed manner. Sharma et al. [40] proposed logarithmic Spiral-Based ABC, which is new feasible variation of ABC. Nayyar et al. [41] reviewed ACO. Ahmad and Choubey [42] discussed about ABC algorithm, and its various types, used for image enhancement in different subdomains of medical imaging. As many of the researcher used PSO, we will discuss only PSO for diagnosis of brain tumor.

For any given problem, there are some ways to evaluate proposed solutions using fitness function. A communication or social network is also defined; each neighbor is assigned to interact with each individual. The population of individuals defined as random guesses at the problem solution is initialized. These individuals are candidate solution and also called as "particle swarm" [37]. Swarm is nothing but a large or dense group of flying insects. Swarms shows flocking behaviors to determine the optimum solution. In PSO, there are two solutions local and global and the algorithm terminates if the global optimal solution is achieved. It consists of three steps: evaluate fitness, update individual and global best, and update velocity and position of every particle.

3.3.5 Particle Swarm Optimization Algorithm

Initialize the parameters

Loop: Iteratively execute till best global optimal solution is achieved.

1. Update Individuals: Particle follows some shortest path to reach a food destination, it is local solution and swarm moves to local best.
2. Update Global Best: Particle keeps track of local and global, specifically global best solution. Global best is shortest path founded so far.

3. Update Velocity: Each individual or particle is associated with velocity, through which it accelerates towards local or global best solution.

Memorize global best, velocity and position of each particle found so far.

End of loop

Output: - The best solution found do far.

3.3.6 Conceptual Framework 2: Applying Swarm Intelligence Based Algorithm for Brain Tumor Diagnosis

Brain tumor diagnosis automated expert system model using swarm intelligence- based algorithm is represented in Figure 3.6. It is similar to

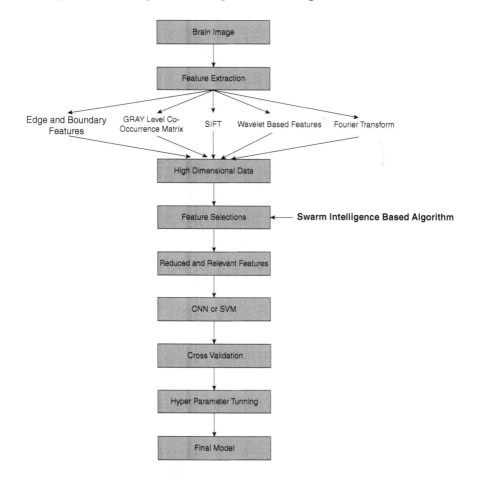

FIGURE 3.6 Swarm intelligence based algorithm for brain tumor diagnosis.

conceptual framework 1; the only difference is instead of evolutionary algorithms, swarm intelligence based algorithms can be applied. As per above discussion PSO can be applied for diagnosis of tumors.

3.4 APPLYING SWARM INTELLIGENCE AND EVOLUTIONARY ALGORITHMS TOGETHER FOR DIAGNOSIS OF BRAIN TUMOR

In this section, we will discuss, how one can apply, evolutionary and swarm intelligence based algorithm together. Evolutionary algorithms can be used for feature selections and hyper tuning can be incorporated with swarm intelligence based algorithm. The figure 3.7 highlights

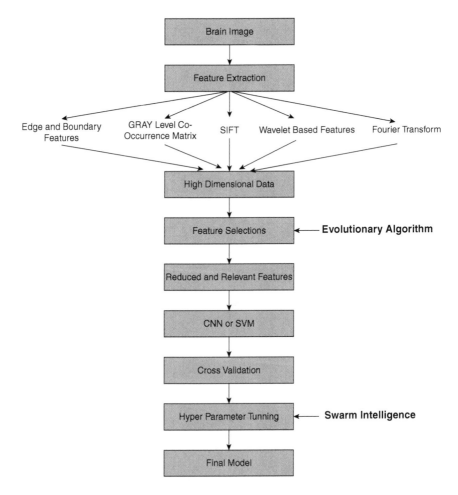

FIGURE 3.7   SI and EA together for diagnosis of brain tumor.

Swarm Intelligence and Evolutionary Algorithm together for diagnosis of brain tumor. The figure 3.7 highlights Swarm Intelligence and Evolutionary Algorithm together for diagnosis of brain tumor. This conceptual framework will give more accuracy as both techniques are working together.

3.5 APPLYING SWARM INTELLIGENCE, EVOLUTIONARY ALGORITHM AND INCORPORATING TOPOLOGICAL DATA ANALYSIS (TDA) FOR BRAIN TUMOR DIAGNOSIS

3.5.1 Topological Data Analysis

Topology is the branch of mathematics, which deals with the shape of the data, shape delivers meaning and meaning provide valuable insights. Points or data in proximity have qualitative features and can give better result. Topology [43] can be applied in healthcare for diagnosis [44] [45] [46] [47]. Machine learning and deep learning works magically with topological data analysis. Using evolutionary algorithms we will get selected reduced features and topological data analysis can be applied over selected features to get meaningful insights that further can be processed using swarm intelligence.

This SWEET (Swarm, Evolutionary and Extraneous Topological Data Analysis) will perform better.

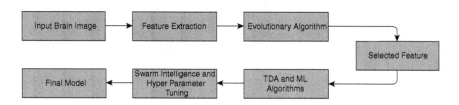

FIGURE 3.8   Incorporating TDA to improve performance of the system.

3.6 CONCLUSION

Computer-aided automated expert system can reduce the overhead of the medical experts, and it can increase the diagnosis accuracy. Though not all NIA are efficient, few of evolutionary algorithms and swarm intelligence-based algorithms provides high efficiency. They can be used for any optimization problems and they provides better solutions with accuracy.

MRI of brain is given as input to intelligent system, conceptual models 1 and 2 uses GA and PSO algorithms to select features. Selected features can be processed further using classifier for prediction. Conceptual model 3 uses a Genetic Algorithm for feature extraction and particle swarm intelligence can be applied along with hyper parameter tuning to get improved performance.

If the topology is incorporated with evolutionary and swarm intelligence, it will form the new model called SWEET. SWEET will not only improved accuracy but also give a performance guarantee.

REFERENCES

[1] Khyati, A. D. (2017). Hybrid nature inspired tumor segmentation using PSO and firefly swarm intelligence. *International Journal of Computer & Mathematical Sciences*, 6(7), 269–275.

[2] Kumar S., Nayyar A., Kumari R. (2019) Arrhenius Artificial Bee Colony Algorithm. In: Bhattacharyya S., Hassanien A., Gupta D., Khanna A., Pan I. (eds) International Conference on Innovative Computing and Communications. Lecture Notes in Networks and Systems, vol 56. Springer, Singapore.

[3] www.bigcloud.io/predicting-a-better-future-with-swarm-intelligence/ (Accessed on 8th April, 2019).

[4] https://www.scmp.com/tech/start-ups/article/2138904/meet-us-start-building-ai-technology-based-collective-human (Accessed on 8th April, 2019).

[5] www.zmescience.com/science/news-science/time-person-year-ai-0432432/ (Accessed on 8th April, 2019).

[6] Barone, L., & While, L. (1999, July). An adaptive learning model for simplified poker using evolutionary algorithms. In *Proceedings of the 1999 Congress on Evolutionary Computation-CEC99 (Cat. No. 99TH8406)* (Vol. 1, pp. 153–160). IEEE.

[7] www.cdc.gov/nchs/fastats/leading-causes-of-death.htm (Accessed on 20th April, 2019).

[8] https://www.healio.com/cardiology/chd-prevention/news/online/%7B3fa64285-7e6e-4068-833e-eb85182aa285%7D/cdc-heart-disease-cancer-leading-causes-of-death-in-2017 (Accessed on 20th April, 2019).

[9] www.who.int/news-room/fact-sheets/detail/cancer (Accessed on 20th April, 2019).

[10] https://www.thebraintumourcharity.org/brain-tumour-diagnosis-treatment/how-brain-tumours-are-diagnosed/brain-tumour-biology/what-is-a-brain-tumour/ (Accessed on 15th November, 2018).

[11] http://braintumor.org/brain-tumor-information/brain-tumor-facts/ (Accessed on 20th April, 2019).

[12] Rajasekaran, K. A., & Gounder, C. C. (2018). Advanced brain tumour segmentation from MRI images. In *High-Resolution Neuroimaging-Basic Physical Principles and Clinical Applications* (pp.83–107). IntechOpen. London.

[13] Kumar, S., Sharma, B., Sharma, V. K., Sharma, H., & Bansal, J. C. (2018). Plant leaf disease identification using exponential spider monkey optimization. *Sustainable Computing: Informatics and Systems*. https://doi.org/10.1016/j.suscom.2018.10.004

[14] Nayyar, A., Garg, S., Gupta, D., & Khanna, A. (2018). Evolutionary computation: Theory and algorithms. In *Advances in Swarm Intelligence for Optimizing Problems in Computer Science* (pp. 1–26). Chapman and Hall/CRC, USA.

[15] Alzubi, J., Nayyar, A., & Kumar, A. (2018, November). Machine learning from theory to algorithms: An overview. *Journal of Physics: Conference Series*, 1142(1), 012012. IOP Publishing.

[16] Satapathy, S. C., & Rajinikanth, V. (2018). Jaya algorithm guided procedure to segment tumor from brain MRI. *Journal of Optimization*, 2018. Vol 2018. DOI: https://doi.org/10.1155/2018/3738049

[17] Kumar, S., Sharma, H., & Jain, S. (2018). In: Advances in Swarm Intelligence for Optimizing Problems in Computer Science, *Genetic Algorithms*, 1(2), 27–52. doi:10.1201/9780429445927-2. Chapman and Hall/CRC.

[18] Vishnulakshmi, K., & SathikRaja, M. (2017). Genetic algorithm based brain tumor detection and segmentation. *International Journal of Innovative Research in Advanced Engineering*, 04(03), 40–47.

[19] Kole, D. K., & Halder, A. (2012). Automatic brain tumor detection and isolation of tumor cells from MRI images. *International Journal of Computer Applications*, 39(16), 26–30.

[20] Sari, M., & Tuna, C. (2018). Prediction of pathological subjects using genetic algorithms. *Computational and Mathematical Methods in Medicine*. Vol.2018. DOI: https://doi.org/10.1155/2018/6154025

[21] Keerthana, T. K., & Xavier, S. (2018, April). An intelligent system for early assessment and classification of brain tumor. In *2018 Second International Conference on Inventive Communication and Computational Technologies (ICICCT)* (pp. 1265–1268). IEEE.

[22] Alalayah, K. M. A., Almasani, S. A. M., Qaid, W. A. A., & Ahmed, I. A. (2018, March). Breast cancer diagnosis based on genetic algorithms and neural networks. *International Journal of Computer Applications*, 180(26), 42–44.

[23] Johnson, P., Vandewater, L., Wilson, W., Maruff, P., Savage, G., Graham, P., ... & Rowe, C. C. (2014). Genetic algorithm with logistic

regression for prediction of progression to Alzheimer's disease. *BMC Bioinformatics, 15*(16), S11.

[24] Nayyar, A., & Singh, R. (2017). Ant colony optimization (ACO) based routing protocols for wireless sensor networks (WSN): A survey. *International Journal* of *Advanced Computer Science* and *Applications, 8*, 148–155.

[25] Nayyar, A., Le, D. N., & Nguyen, N. G. (Eds.). (2018). *Advances in Swarm Intelligence for Optimizing Problems in Computer Science.* CRC Press., USA.

[26] Nayyar, A., & Nguyen, N. G. (2018). Introduction to swarm intelligence. In *Advances in Swarm Intelligence for Optimizing Problems in Computer Science* (pp. 53–78). Chapman and Hall/CRC, USA.

[27] Kamble, T., & Rane, P. (2013, May). Brain tumor segmentation using swarm intelligence approach. *International Journal of Scientific & Engineering Research, 4*(5), 716–719.

[28] Bonabeau, E., Marco, D. D. R. D. F., Dorigo, M., & Theraulaz, G. (1999). *Swarm intelligence: From natural to artificial systems* (No. 1). Oxford university press United Kingdom (U.K).

[29] Kennedy, J., & Eberhart, R. (1995, November). Particle swarm optimization (PSO). In *Proceeding IEEE International Conference on Neural Networks* (pp. 1942–1948). Perth, Australia.

[30] Banchpalliwar, R., & Salankar, S. Diagnosis of Brain Tumor Through MRI Image Processing using Clustering with Optimization Technique. International Journal of Innovative Research in Computer and Communication Engineering 4(4), 5303–5310.

[31] Zamani, H., & Nadimi-Shahraki, M. H. (2016, October). Swarm intelligence approach for breast cancer diagnosis. *International Journal of Computer Applications, 151*(1), 40–44.

[32] Punidha, R., Sakthivel, S., Nehru, V., & Gunasundari, C. (2017). Segmentation of brain tumor MRI based on particle swarm optimization. *International Journal of Pure and Applied Mathematics, 116*(13), 1–7.

[33] Gunavathi, C., & Premalatha, K. (2014). A comparative analysis of swarm intelligence techniques for feature selection in cancer classification. *The Scientific World Journal.* Vol 2014. DOI: http://dx.doi.org/10.1155/2014/693831

[34] Adithyan, T. A., Sharma, V., Gururaj, B., & Thirumalai, C. (2017, May). Nature inspired algorithm. In *2017 International Conference on Trends in Electronics and Informatics (ICEI)* (pp. 1131–1134). IEEE.

[35] Muslim, M. A., Rukmana, S. H., Sugiharti, E., Prasetiyo, B., & Alimah, S. (2018, March). Optimization of C4. 5 algorithm-based particle swarm optimization for breast cancer diagnosis. *Journal of Physics: Conference Series, 983*(1), 012063. IOP Publishing.

[36] Selvanayaki, K. (2013). Intelligent brain tumor tissue segmentation from magnetic resonance image (MRI) using meta heuristic algorithms. *Journal of Global Research in Computer Science, 4*(2), 13–20.

[37] Selvi, V., & Umarani, R. (2010). Comparative analysis of ant colony and particle swarm optimization techniques. *International Journal of Computer Applications, 5*(4), 1–6.

[38] Durbhaka, G. K., Selvaraj, B., & Nayyar, A. (2019). Firefly swarm: Metaheuristic swarm intelligence technique for mathematical optimization. In *Data Management, Analytics and Innovation* (pp. 457–466). Springer, Singapore.

[39] Nayyar, A., Puri, V., & Suseendran, G. (2019). Artificial bee colony optimization—population-based meta-heuristic swarm intelligence technique. In *Data Management, Analytics and Innovation* (pp. 513–525). Springer, Singapore.

[40] Sharma, S., Kumar, S., & Nayyar, A. (2018, August). Logarithmic spiral based local search in artificial bee colony algorithm. In *International Conference on Industrial Networks and Intelligent Systems* (pp. 15–27). Springer, Cham.

[41] Nayyar, A., & Singh, R. (2016, March). Ant colony optimization—computational swarm intelligence technique. In *2016 3rd International Conference on Computing for Sustainable Global Development (INDIACom)* (pp. 1493–1499). IEEE.

[42] Ahmad, R., & Choubey, N. S. (2018). Review on image enhancement techniques using biologically inspired artificial bee colony algorithms and its variants. In *Biologically Rationalized Computing Techniques for Image Processing Applications* (pp. 249–271). Springer, Cham.

[43] Carlsson, G. (2009). Topology and data. *Bulletin of the American Mathematical Society, 46*(2), 255–308.

[44] Nicolau, M., Levine, A. J., & Carlsson, G. (2011). Topology based data analysis identifies a subgroup of breast cancers with a unique mutational profile and excellent survival. *Proceedings of the National Academy of Sciences, 108*(17), 7265–7270.

[45] Nielson, J. L., Paquette, J., Liu, A. W., Guandique, C. F., Tovar, C. A., Inoue, T., ... & Lum, P. Y. (2015). Topological data analysis for discovery in preclinical spinal cord injury and traumatic brain injury. *Nature Communications, 6*, 8581.

[46] Li, L., Cheng, W. Y., Glicksberg, B. S., Gottesman, O., Tamler, R., Chen, R., ... & Dudley, J. T. (2015). Identification of type 2 diabetes subgroups through topological analysis of patient similarity. *Science Translational Medicine, 7*(311), 311ra174–311ra174.

[47] Lockwood, S., & Krishnamoorthy, B. (2014). Topological features in cancer gene expression data. In *Pacific Symposium on Biocomputing Co-Chairs* (pp. 108–119).

Swarm Intelligence and Evolutionary Algorithms for Diabetic Retinopathy Detection

Sachin Bhandari and Radhakrishna Rambola

Department of Computer Engineering, SVKM's NMIMS (Deemed to be university), Mukesh Patel School of Technology Management & Engineering, Shirpur, India

Rajani Kumari

Department of Computer Application and IT, JECRC University, Jaipur, India

4.1 INTRODUCTION

In the last few decades, it has been observed that diabetes is rising at an extremely high pace across the world. The number of diabetic patients is increasing exponentially, which is a challenge for the healthcare sector. According to the annual World Health Organization survey, diabetes is on a continuous growth. Diabetes is a disease which is the starting point of various health issues. Macrovascular variations are the major complications that result because of diabetes, e.g. diabetic retinopathy (DR), renal and heart ailments [1].

A latest survey states that diabetes is the fifth dangerous disease type that does not have effective cure and measures [2,3]. DR is a very common problem in diabetes. It is actually the major cause of blindness in the patients. One survey says that more than 75% of the population with DR belong to developing countries, hence the complications cannot be handled due to lack of treatment facilities. Those having DR probably suffer blindness [4] because until the time it can be recognized by an individual the changes in retina reach an extent such that it cannot be curable.

4.1.1 Classification of Diabetic Retinopathy

DR is a micro-angiopathy that shows features of microvascular occlusion and leakage, and it is important to be familiar with the signs of occlusion and leakage in the retina to understand the pathogenesis and signs of DR. DR pathogenesis comprises capillaropathy, haematological changes, micro-vascular occlusion [1]. So, what happens to blood vessels in the presence of diabetes, high blood sugar causes several things to occur in the blood vessels, there capillaropathy where the blood vessels walls degenerate, haematological changes where deformity of blood cells occurs and thickening of the blood happens and finally microvascular occlusion, causes irregular blood flow and decreased oxygen. Classification of DR are given as follows:

1. Non-proliferative DR(NPDR) (background DR)

2. Maculopathy

3. Pre-proliferative

4. Proliferative

1. Non-proliferative Diabetic Retinopathy
The signs of background or NPDR are microaneurysms, retinal hae-morrhages, macular edema and hard exudates. DR stages can be identified on the basis of DR features and severity [5]. NPDR can be further classified into three categories: early NPDR, moderate NPDR, severe NPDR. These stages of NPDR are described as follows:

(a) Early NPDR: It contains microaneurysms with hard exudates and haemorrhage or without them. Almost 50% of the diabetic patients have minimum [6], i.e. mild NPDR symptoms.

(b) Moderate NPDR: In this stage many microaneurysms with hard exudates and haemorrhage are present. A study reveal that 16% patient of non-proliferative DR are probably convert into proliferative DR (PDR) within a year [7].

(c) Severe NPDR: These type of NPDR represents by following characteristics [1]:

    i. In four quadrants multiple haemorrhages and microaneurysms presents.

    ii. Two or more quadrants full of bleeding (venous)

    iii. In minimum one quadrant intraretinal microvascular abnormalities present.

In DR the first stage is NPDR. In NPDR the blood vessels of the retina begin to weaken causing tiny lumps called micro-aneurysms to swell out from the walls of the vessels. In this stage, very mild symptoms may be felt or there may be no symptoms at all. Gradually, the blood vessels start getting blocked and transport less and less blood. Some areas are stared of oxygen and begin to send signals to the retina to create new blood vessels. Hence, it is essential for a diabetic patient to have regular check-ups to ensure early diagnosis and treatment. NPDR will be converted in to PDR within one year, there will be approximately 50% probability of this [7].

2. Maculopathy
Any edema hard exudate or ischemia which involves the fovea is termed diabetic maculopathy, and this is the most common cause of vision impairment in diabetes, especially those with type 2 diabetes as there are few different types of Maculopathy is their focal in one area diffuse spread all around ischemic or clinically significant macular edema[1]. Here we discuss clinically significant macular edema because it is the clinically significant. It is observed in an image of a blurry macula with some dot haemorrhages with hard exudates near, hence a thickened macula is actually easier to detect on OCT.

3. Pre-Proliferative DR (PPDR)
Background DR that shows sign of imminent proliferative disease is called pre-proliferative DR (PPDR). Clinically signs indicate progressive retinal ischemia and the signs include:

    i. Cotton wool spots (soft exudates)

    ii. Intraretinal microvascular abnormalities (IRMA)

    iii. Other changes like venous and retinal arterial changes and dark blot haemorrhages

The risk of actually progressing to PDR depends on the number of lesions seen on the retina, and you can actually have proliferative disease in one eye and pre-proliferative in other [8]. It contains three abnormalities that are intraretinal microvascular abnormalities (IRMA), arterial changes, dark blood haemorrhages.

Intraretinal micro vascular abnormalities (IRMA): They are fine irregular red lines that runs from arteries to the venous. When tiny changes in the vasculature are seen, it is a clear indication that it's actually free of DR and may progress to proliferative venous changes, which are also common in proof relief DR and include symptoms like dilated and tortuous veins. Looping blood vessels bleeding is there where you can see the little bead-like structures where the vessels begin to start to look like little beads and sausage-like segmentation where the vessels look like a string of sausages.

Arterial Changes: These changes in pre proliferative DR include peripheral neuron of the arteries something called silver wiring, where it looks like silver wire that has been inserted into the artery itself and then complete obliteration where it is actually missing and completely blocked.

Dark blood haemorrhages: These are retinal haemorrhages found in the middle retinal layers, and they are exactly as described—dark blood haemorrhages bleeding into the retina.

4. Proliferative Diabetic Retinopathy (PDR)

PDR is an advanced form; DR progressive circulation to the retina is affected due to which new blood vessels begin to grow into the retina and into the gel-like fluid called vitreous that fills the central posterior segment or cavity of the eye. These blood vessels are thin and delicate, and may leak blood into the vitreous causing clouding of vision [1].

The macula is the small region of the retina that is responsible for sharp detailed central vision. When the fluid leaks into the macula, it causes the macula to swell resulting in blurred vision. As the retina gets damaged, scar tissue is formed and pressure builds up in the rear chamber. This could result in damage to the optic nerve at the same time; as scar tissue shrinks it pulls at the retina and a portion of the retina may break loose from the back of the eye, this is called "retinal detachment," which results in gradual loss of vision and ultimately blindness.

The classification of PDR contains neovascularisation, rubeosis, neo-vascularization at a disc as signs:

(a) Neovascularization (NV): It is stated as a typical emergence of new blood vessels that usually emerges on the internal surfaces of retina [1]. This is caused by angiogenic growth factor increased by hypoxic retinal tissues in an attempt to revascularization of the hypoxic retina, so there is lack of oxygen in these vascular endothelial growth factors and they create new blood vessels and neovascularization. The problem with the new blood vessels is that they are irregular, they are not formed well, they are fragile and then they burst and leak. The sign of neovascularisation is mottled mess of very fine blood vessels.

(b) Rubeosis: It occurs with PDR and rubeosis appears as neovascular-ization but it is neovascularization at iris and this is definitely not a normal state of affairs.

(c) Neovascularization disc (NVD): The term NVD in a patient file that stands for neovascularization elsewhere and that means neo-vascularization occurring somewhere in the retina not at the disc.

4.1.2 Swarm Optimization and Evolutionary Algorithms

In swarm optimization, birds, bees, fish and ants, all of these creatures are evolved methods of amplifying their intelligence by syncing together, thinking together in systems, this is why flock in fish school and bees swarm they are together than alone [9]. Actually, there is no discussion about crowd sourcing like humans do by taking votes in polls and surveys, there is a discussion about forming real-time systems with feed-back loops, so deeply interconnected that a new intelligence forms and emergent intelligence with its own personality and intellect. There is a discussion about forming a hive mind, biologist call this swarm intelligence and it's a natural step in the evolution of most social species.

A brain is a system of neurons so deeply connected that intelligence forms a swarm, which is a system of brain, swarm is a brain of brains and it can be in any individual. For example, there are group of large number of honey bees and they have a very difficult problem to solve; they need to find a new home to move into that, a new home could be hollow log of a hole in the side of a building or anything. It sounds like a simple problem, but this is connected to life or death decision that could impact the survival of the colony for generations, so to solve this problem the colony sends out hundreds of scout bees which search a 30 square mile area and find dozens of candidate sites. That's the easy part; the hard part is that they need to pick the best possible solution from all the options that they have discovered [10].

Honey bees have a tiny brain which is smaller than a grain of sand and has less than a million neurons; human have 85 billion neurons, so however smart humans think honey bees have the intelligence equal to the human intelligence divide by 85,000. Honey bees are very discriminating house hunters as they need to find a new home that's large enough to store the honey they need for winter, is ventilated well enough to stay cool in the summer, is insulated well enough to stay warm in cold nights, is protected from the rain, is near a good source of clean water, and of course is well located near good sources of pollen: this is a complex multivariable problem and to optimize survival the bees need to pick the best possible solution across all the competing constraints and they do it remarkably.

Biologists have shown that honeybees picked the best possible solution over 80% of the time, however, if a human CEO needs to find the perfect location for a new factory, he or she would face a similarly complex problem and it would be very difficult to pick the optimal solution, and yet honey bees can do it. A honey bee has a brain so tiny that it cannot even conceive the problem, but when they think together in a system they can solve it accurately; they can rival a human brain. How do they do this? They do it by forming a swarm intelligence, a brain of brains that combines the knowledge and wisdom and insight and intuition of the group and converges on optimized decisions [11].

Honeybees do everything by vibrating their bodies; biologists calls this waggle dance because for humans it looks like bees are dancing, but in reality they are generating the signals that represent their support for the various home sites under consideration and by combining these signals the bees engage in a multidirectional tug of war pushing and pulling on the decision until they find that one solution that can be best agreed upon. It is usually the optimal solution and unlike us humans the bees don't entrench, don't fall into gridlock, don't settle for a bad solution that nobody's happy with, instead they find the solution that's best for the group as whole. Swarms are flexible and dynamic reviewing. Why humans amplify our intelligence now if birds, bees and fish can form a brain of brains. Why can't people do it? Swarm turns in to artificial super experts who can make more accurate, predictions, decisions evaluations, and forecasts. This is about the natural swarm. Over the last few years, we have been modelling how swarms like this amplify the intelligence of groups and using those models to create the algorithms and interfaces that enable humans to form similar swarms online [12]. Here swarm optimization and evolutionary algorithms are used to create the models for the detection of DR. This chapter contains the features of DR, models for DR, and approaches for detection of DR.

4.1.3 Objectives and Contributions

Diabetes increases day by day in a living being, the mellitus results of diabetes turn into micro-vasculature which causes DR. As the DR increases by time, it causes complete vision loss. For efficient completion of DR practises, it is necessary to identify the variations and morphological changes in micro-aneurysms, optic disk, retinal blood vessels, hard exudates, soft exudates, haemorrhages, etc. These types of identifications are complicated and require computer-aided diagnostic system (CAD) by which the DR may be identified earlier. The aim of this chapter is to discuss and analyse the CAD systems that are designed and implemented for effective identification of DR.

The main objective of the study is to focus on the traditional and latest approaches of CAD systems by which DR can be identified in early stages efficiently. Here the discussion and analysis of number of existing literatures represent DR CAD systems.

The approaches discussed here are evolutionary approaches that contain particle swarm optimization (PSO), genetic algorithm (GA), ant colony optimization (ACO) and bee colony optimization. These evolutionary computing approaches can play an important role for optimizing DR-CAD components like pre-processing, feature extraction, dimensional reduction, feature selection, clustering and classification.

The learning objectives of the chapter are as follows:

(a) Recognize the importance of DR as a public problem.

(b) Discuss DR as a leading cause of blindness in developed countries.

(c) Identify the risk factors for DR.

(d) Describe and distinguish between the stages of DR.

(e) Understand the role of swarm intelligence and evolutionary computing approaches for the prevention of vision loss and early detection of DR.

4.2 FEATURE OF DIABETIC RETINOPATHY

These features represent the deficiency caused by the diabetes disease. It is observed that there are main problems in retinal damage which is to be mentioned below. Table 4.1 represents the characteristics, colour, shape and volume affected by the following abnormalities.

4.2.1 Microaneurysms

This is one of the signs of NPDR; they are localized out pouching of the capillary wall spreading out and in a certain area thickening up and moving in an outward direction so that these microaneurysms can leak plasma into the retina because the blood retinal barrier is

TABLE 4.1   Characterization of various abnormalities based on colour, shape and volume.

Types of Abnormalities	Characteristics	Colour	Shape	Volume affected
Microaneurysms	These are tiny aneurysms which causes swelling in the side of blood vessels	Red spot	Small circular	Small
Haemorrhages	These have a flame-like appearance or they can be intra retinal and located in the middle layers of the retina	Bright red	Not defined	Large
Hard exudates	Hard exudates are caused by retinal edema and develop at the junction of normal and swollen retina	Yellow	Circular	Large
Soft exudates	Vessel occlusion as opposed to hard exudates which result from vascular leakage	Yellowish white	Not defined	Large
Neo vascularization	Emergence of new blood vessel on the internal surface of retina.	Red	Not defined	Large
Macular edema	It causes leakage of fluid or solutes around the macula	Not defined	Roundish	Large

broken down or thrombosed and there are some little out-pouching dots of microaneurysms coming out of these tiny little blood vessels. The signs include tiny little red dots initially temporal to the fovea which are the earliest signs of DR, but they are hard to see when you are looking at the fundus and actually more obvious during fundus fluorescein and geography. It is of the eye that had a fundus fluorescein angiogram and their tiny little specks are microaneurysms. The changes in retinal blood vessels formed microaneurysms [8]. It is in round shape and it has dark red spots, temporarily called macula.

4.2.2 Haemorrhages

It's quite easy to get confused with dot haemorrhages which are more easily seen on the retina because they are actually larger and quite similar. The retinal haemorrhages and heritage can appear actually either in the retinal nerve fibre layer and these have a flame-like appearance or they can be intra-retinal and located in the middle layers of the retina and have a red-dot blot appearance, so these dot blot haemorrhages can be a larger version of microaneurysms that they look similar on the retina. The leakage in blood vessels causes haemorrhages [13]. They look like a red spot, having non-uniform margin with varying density.

4.2.3 Hard Exudates

Hard exudates are caused by retinal edema and develop at the junction of normal and swollen retina. They are made up of lipoproteins and lipid-filled macrophages and are waxy yellow in appearance with distinct margins. They are usually arranged in clumps or ring shape around the retina and are often surrounding microaneurysms. When the leakage stops occurring in the retina, these can reabsorb but it can take months or years [13,14].

4.2.4 Soft Exudates

Hard exudates are made up of lipids and they are yellow in colour and often found close to the macula. They have distinct margins and result from blood vessel leakage. Cotton wool spots on the other hand are made up of axonal debris and they are more prominent around the optic nerve, where the nerve fibre lays the cast and are lighter and coloured light yellow or white as opposed to the darker yellow of hard exudates. Cotton wall spots are sort of billowy-like clouds that do not have distinct margins, which result from vessel occlusion as opposed to hard exudates which result from vascular leakage.

In general, CWS occurs because of the occlusion of arteriole [15]. The reduced blood flow to the retina results into ischemia of the retinal nerve fibre layer (RNFL) that eventually influences the axoplasmic flow and thus accumulates axoplasmic debris across the retinal ganglion cell axons. Such accumulation can be visualized like fluffy white lesions in the RNFL, which is commonly known as CWS [15,16].

4.2.5 Neo-Vascularization

This is caused by angiogenic growth factor increased by hypoxic retinal tissues in an attempt to revascularization of the hypoxic retina, so what happens is that there is lack of oxygen in these. Vascular endothelial growth factors kick in and they create new blood vessels and neovascularization. The problem with the new blood vessels is that they are irregular, not formed well, are fragile, and then they burst and leak[17].

4.2.6 Macular Edema

This is caused by extensive capillary leakage or leakage from microaneurysms and dilated capillaries, so what happens is fluid accumulates in the inner retinal layers and if the fluid accumulates under the fovea it can eventually develop a sea storied appearance and is called "sisterhood macular edema." You can observe the retinal thickening and the cyst with space in the OCT scans generally, in which surely the bottom part shows a fundus fluorescein angiogram of a patient with macular edema, it will typical a flower-like pattern where the cysts fill up with fluorescein and have this little roundish appearance. Actually it is a swollen part of the eye retina, it occurs due to problems of anomalous retinal capillaries [18,19].

4.3 DETECTION OF DIABETIC RETINOPATHY BY APPLYING SWARM INTELLIGENCE AND EVOLUTIONARY ALGORITHMS

There are many mathematical models and a number of different analytical approaches has been proposed and developed for DR. The traditional approaches are found limited so there will be consideration of complex features, many computational complexities and many solutions presence, etc. For DR and related problems, there will be some approaches of evolutionary computing, which are based on the concepts of natural phenomenon and human centric which drives an affinity, effectiveness and an idea for treatment, attention across the society and industry. There will be some efforts on exploring its efficiency towards DR, so there will be description of different types of Evolutionary Computing algorithms for DR.

An evolutionary computing (EC) approaches are based on natural phenomenon and it is observed that EC are most effective procedure to build a model because these are primarily evolved from the concept of natural bird's quality. There are number of approaches and models built for DR detection and diagnoses that are based on EC algorithms. There will be consideration of complex feature, different solutions, computational problem and traditional approaches are found confined, so to handle these different problems recently EC and swarm intelligence approaches are used [9]. Here a discussion of different efforts taken by EC approaches towards DR. In this given context we explore the EC algorithms for DR processes.

4.3.1 Genetic Algorithm

The GA is a method for solving both constrained and unconstrained optimization problems that is based on natural selection, the process that drives biological evolution. GA is a powerful tool for solving large-scale design optimization problems [9]. The research interests in GAs lie in both its theory and applications. GA is a type of meta-heuristic search and optimization algorithm inspired by Darwin's principle of natural selection. The central idea of natural selection is survival of the fittest. Through the process of natural selection, organisms adapt to optimize their chances for survival in a given environment.

The general procedures of a GA include:

1. Create a population of random individuals

2. Evaluate each individual's fitness

3. Select individuals to be parents

4. Produce children

5. Evaluate children

6. Repeat 3 to 5 until a solution with satisfied fitness is found or some predetermined number of generations is met.

To yield better solutions higher fitness value signifies higher probability of a chromosome to take participate in the next generation. Offsprings are built using GA based on estimated fitness value, mutation probability (P_m) and crossover probability (P_c). Implementing the population generation continues till the criteria is reached and optimal solution is obtained. Considering robustness of GA, it has been used in an array of applications, including DR, where it is primarily suggested for feature selection and as the enhancement model for classifiers. The following sections discuss the key literatures exploiting GA for DR model development. The methods and salient feature used by the authors for research are shown in Table 4.2.

a) Feature in fundus

Osareh et al. [20] suggests a computational intelligence techniques-based model which takes images of retinopathy as input and identifies

TABLE 4.2 Performance measures of GA based models

Author	Method	Salient feature
Osareh et al. [20]	Neural network, GA	Gabor filters, retinal exudates
Rashid et al. [21]	Fuzzy C-means, GA	Fuzzy histogram equalization
Naluguru et al. [22]	Neural network, GA	Bacterial foraging algorithm
Karegowda et al. [23]	GA- correlation based feature selection, BPNN	Feature selection, Decision tree
Ganesan et al. [24]	GA, SVM	Trace transformation
Nirosha et al. [25]	GA, Adaptive Neuro Fuzzy Inference system	Low-cost CAD model
Santos et al. [26]	GA, SVM	Optical coherence tomography (OCT)
Quellec et al. [27]	GA, Powell's direction set descent.	Local lesion template matching, optimal wavelets transform.
Akram et al. [28]	GA, SVM	GMM, eeightestimation
Lee et al. [29]	GA	Fundus auto-fluorescence (FAF), age-related macular degeneration (AMD)
Hung et al. [30]	RIS system, TRDD system, GA	Tractional retinal detachment

exudates pathologies automatically. The segmentation of images is done by fuzzy C-means clustering. These segmentations contain pre-processing steps, i.e. contrast enhancement and colour normalization. To classify the segmented region, they need to set some feature initially, such as strength, size, colour etc. The GA is used to learn the given features to rank them and to identify the subset and to identify the subset which gives the accurate classification results.

Rashid et al. [21] proposed an efficient screening model for exudates detection in fundus images which are compatible to real-time applications. In this automated model, fuzzy C-means techniques are used in collaboration with morphological techniques, to improve the robustness of blood vessel and optic disc detection. There are different set of initial features considered to discriminate exudates regions from other segmented regions such as compactness of the region, region size, length of the perimeter of the region, region edge strength, mean value inside the region, mean value outside the region, standard deviation of mean values inside and outside the region and region mean filter responses.

b) Segmentation of Retinal Lesions

EC techniques for segmentation are presented by Naluguru et al. [22]. It is a type of feature extraction technique which contains blood vessel segmentation in automatic DR. They are using GA with SVM and Bacterial Foraging Algorithm (BFA) to extract the blood vessels, texture, optic disc and entropies from the retina. It involves in segmentation after that it will extract the features from the images based on bifurcation points, texture, entropy then moves to statistical feature extraction. After statistical feature extraction, authors use GA and BFO with neural network to classify the images into three categories, normal, NPDR and PDR, and then find the best classifier for retinal lesion and grade them into gentle moderate and extreme.

c) Feature extraction of exudates

Karegowda et al. [23] developed a CAD system or automated system that can effectively classify the retinopathy images and improve the diabetic screening program. They have used a BPNN (Back Propagation Neural Network) model to classify the images and detect exudates. That model further improved by using two methods that are DT (Decision tree) and GA-CFS (GA correlation-based feature selection).

Ganesan et al. [24] formed an efficient model for feature extraction of exudates. First, they have taken retinal images dataset, then perform pre-processing, and then visualize a model based on Trace Transform function. This model will do the feature ranking and selection and then classify them by using SVM and PNN (probabilistic neural network) and optimize that with GA.

d) Segmentation of exudates

A very effective CAD model has been developed by Nirosha et al. [25] in which author has used GA and ANFIS (Adaptive Neuro Fuzzy Inference System) together to classify and detectabnormalities of DR. Santos et al. [26] focused on OCT (optical coherence tomography) data for effective classification using SVM classifier. The classification is totally based on OCT data. In the proposed approach, different materials and methods are used like data gathering and OCT data model based on logarithmic of linear spaces. Perform discrimination between eyes of healthy peoples and diabetic patients, at last measures parameter choice through GA heuristic search. After parameter choice validation of the selected data model for SVM, discrimination is performed.

e) Microaneurysms detection

Quellec et al. [27] proposed an automatic detection model to test micro-aneurysms in retina images. For microaneurysms model validation, a multimodal photographic image database is used to find the mean and standard deviation of the pixel. The proposed approach represents template matching in the wavelet domainthese wavelet domains consider template matching, adaptation in the wavelet domain and moving windows approach. Overall learning procedure will be follow as the images of the learning dataset then form a wavelet transform using wavelet filter, these wavelets transformed the images and compute the distance of the model.. It will follow by grid search with a particular threshold and calculate the efficiency. This proposed model learning procedure contains model parameter selection, subset learning and wavelet learning. It will efficiently detect microaneurysms. Akram et al. [28] in this author proposed a hybrid model for classification using support vector machine and GMM classify region as micro aneurysms or non-microaneurysms. To improve the accuracy author applied GA with weight estimation for classification that increases the accuracy. This approach includes pre-processing which can extract feasible Region of interest.

f) Segmentation of blood vessel

Lee et al. [29] present a segmentation method to preserve interest of features. Author has used fundus auto-fluorescence (FAF) images, which is used to show segmentation then GA plays an important role, in this GA prone to inter and intra observer variability. Here classification and segmentation is done by using GA quantification and this automatic quantification for determining AMD diagnosis and disease progression. They are identifying hypo-fluorescent GA regions from retinal vessel structures. Hung et al. [30] proposed a system of segmentation to detect blood vessels from retinal images, dark spots, bright spots, etc. Author proposed a tractional retinal detachment diagnosis system based on retinal images that can provide impressive results in segmentation of bright spots and dark spots. The system they have made is RIS (retinopathy image segmentation) that correctly segments all the regions. In this to identify the most appropriate results of the parameters resides in RIS system; author has used genetic-based parameter detector—retinopathy image segmentation method (GBPD-RIS). Another system they have developed is called TRDD (tractional retinal detachment disease), which is based on diabetic patient's retinal images. The TRDD contains three steps: first analysis of GLCM (Gray-level Co-occurrence matrix), BFM and GBPD-TRDD system. The co-occurrence texture statistics contain different features like contrast, dissimilarity, correlation, inverse difference moment. The methods and salient feature used by the authors for research are shown in table 4.2.

4.3.2 Particle Swarm Optimization

A particle is a small localized object to which several physical or chemical properties such as volume or mass can be ascribed. Swarm is a collection of something that move somewhere in large numbers, e.g. flock, crowd, flood, etc. Optimization is the action of making the best or most effective use of a situation or resource [31], e.g. minimizing the total travel time from one city to other. PSO is a population-based stochastic technique inspired by social behaviour of bird flocking or fish schooling. The scenario of PSO is that, a group of birds are randomly searching food in an area [32]. There is only one piece of food in the area being searched. All the birds do not know where food resides, but they know how far the food presents. So, using the best strategy to find food, the effective one is to follow the bird which is nearest to the food. In PSO, each single solution is a "bird" in the search space called "particle". All of particles have fitness values which are evaluated by the fitness function to be optimized, and have velocities which direct the flying of the particles. The particles fly through the problem space by following the current optimum particles [33]. In this study, the PSO is used for detection of DR. The methods and salient feature used by the authors for research are shown in Table 4.3.

a) Retinal images feature extraction

Anitha et al. [34] compare the performance of GA and PSO and prove that both the techniques yield optimal solutions with different strategies and computational efforts. IT is used for feature selection in retinal images. They classify the retinal images in to four classes named central retinal vein occlusion (CRVO), choroid neo-vascularisation membrane (CNVO), NPDR, and central serious retinopathy. There is a methodology of the automated retinal classification in which retinal images database is used for experiment. Feature extraction of retinal images can be done by GA and PSO then classified using SOFM based classification. The selected features in PSO are area, perimeter, skewness, and correlation and inverse difference moments and in GA the features selected are area, perimeter, kurtosis, correlation and contrast. Balakrishnan et al. [35] proposed a hybrid model for classification and feature

TABLE 4.3   Performance measures of PSO based models

Author	Method	Salient feature
Anitha et al. [34]	SOFM Neural Network, PSO, GA	Central retinal vein occlusion (CRVO), choroidal neo-vascularization membrane (CNVO)
Balakrishnan et al. [35]	PSO, SVM, differential evolution (DE) algorithms	Histogram of orient gradient (HOG), complete local binary pattern (CLBP)
Ravivarma et al. [36]	PSO, SVM, FCM	Hyperbolic median filter
Sreejini et al. [37]	Retina vessels, PSO	Optic disc, Fovea, multiscale matched filter
Sreejini et al. [38]	PSO, ETDRS	Mathematical morphology
Devasia et al. [39]	PSO, DRION database	Histogram, localized optic disc

extraction from retinal images. Channel extraction and median filter areused for pre-processing of retinal images. After pre-processing of images, authors used histogram of oriented gradient (HOG) with complete local binary pattern (CLBP) to perform feature selection. In this model, PSO is used to optimize the results.

b) Exudates segmentation

An efficient system is designed and implemented for detection of exudates in colour fundus images using image processing techniques. Ravivarma et al. [36] present a novel approach to achieve efficient identification of exudates in low-quality retinal images. Hyperbolic median filter is used for pre-processing then segmentation is done by using fuzzy C-means clustering algorithm. The features like colour, size, and texture extract from segmentation of images. After segmentation the features are optimized through PSO and then classified by SVM. Sreejini et al. [37] implement a multiscale matched filter for retina vessel segmentation using PSO algorithm. The performance of multiscale matched filter is much better then single scale matched filter. This approach removes the noise suppression feature of multiscale filter. For finding optimal filter parameters of the multiscale Gaussian matched filter author used PSO.

c) Segmentation of blood vessels

Sreejini et al. [38] developed a model which is unsupervised in nature and can classify the severity of diabetic macular edema in colour fundus images. The early detection of macula for the treatment of DR is necessary and to achieve this author use PSO. Hassan et al. proposed an approach for enhancing segmentation and extract the vasculature on retinal fundus images using PSO.

d) Optic disc segmentation

A histogram-based approach is developed by Devasia et al. [39] in collaboration with PSO to identify optical disc. Optical disc detection is a major problem in DR image datasets. By this approach author get higher positive correlation which possess by localized optic disc centres.

4.3.3 Ant Colony Optimization

Ants have inspired a number of methods and techniques among which the most studied and the most successful is the general-purpose optimization technique known as ACO. ACO takes inspiration from the foraging behaviour of some ant species [40]. These ants deposit pheromone on the ground in order to mark some favourable path that should be followed by other members of the colony. The pheromone is a chemical substance released into the environment by an animal, especially a mammal or an insect, affecting the behaviour or physiology of others of its species. Ants navigate from nest to food source, ants are blind. Shortest path is discovered via pheromone trails. Each ant moves randomly and pheromone is deposited on the path. More pheromone on path increases probability of path being followed [36]. The methods and salient feature used by the authors for research are shown in Table 4.4.

a) Segmentation of blood vessel

Bajčeta et al. [41] developed a model for segmentation of blood vessels in which they have applied ACO in fundus images and ACO perform feature extraction. Hooshyar et al. [42] proposed a mathematical model in which they have used Eigen values of hessian matrix and Gabor filter bank to extract the features from retinal images. An approach for classification is developed by using fuzzy c-means and ACO. Asad et al. [43] proposed an approach and ensure an improvement of the ant clustering-based segmentation. The first approach is developed with the help of new heuristic function of the ACO algorithm. The second approach is based on global update mechanism of ACO. They have compared the proposed system

TABLE 4.4   Performance measures of ACO based models

Author	Method	Salient feature
Bajčeta et al. [41]	ACO	Blood vessel segmentation
Hooshyar et al. [42]	ACO, Fuzzy clustering	Eigen value of hessian matrix, Gabon filter.
Asad et al. [43]	ACO	Heuristic function
Asad et al. [44]	Enhanced ACO	Feature pol technique
Pereira et al. [45]	Unsupervised model, Image processing, ACO	Multiagent system, exudates
Karthikeyan et al. [46]	FP growth model, ACO	Association rule mining
Kavitha et al. [47]	ACO	OTSU method, optic disc, macula
Arnay et al. [48]	ACO, OPTIC CUP segmentation model	Heuristic function, intensity gradient, vessel's curvature

with various traditional systems of blood vessel segmentation. Proposed approach followed by phases like pre-processing phase in which extraction of green channel of retinal image is perform then the linear transformation of its intensity to cover the whole intensity range [0, 255], then removal of the central light reflex from it. Next phase will be ACS-based segmentation and at last applying median filter of size 3*3 to remove all remaining isolated pixels. Asad et al. [44] proposed an improved model against previous one. In this proposed work, author try to achieve early detection by automatic segmentation of retinal blood vessels in retinal images that is also called a two-class problem. They proposed two improvements in previous approaches, first including features to the feature pool which was further used for classification, in second improvement they combined probability theory based heuristic function with ACO and remove the old Euclidean distance method used in previous.

b) Segmentation of exudates

For early detection of exudates, Pereira et al. [45] proposed an unsupervised method with ACO for exudates segmentation. They have taken green plane images given to median filter background estimation then normalize them and place a double threshold and perform candidate selection. Analyse the exudates with ACO algorithm, then ACO presents edges enhancement. Karthikeyan et al. [46] proposed a new algorithm-based approach in which they used association rule mining in collaboration with enhanced FP growth algorithm which is similar to ACO. The algorithm used in this approach is also called as CACO, i.e. Continuous Ant colony Optimization algorithm for segmentation of exudates.

c) Segmentation of optic disc

Kavitha et al. [47] classify optic disc and macula in normal and abnormal classes. They have used ACO-based method for macula and optic disc detection. The radius of optic disc and distance between the centres of optic disc is used as a feature in this approach. The approach is followed by input of the images for pre-processing. Pre-processed images are given for optic disc detection by ACO and further Macula is detection done by Otsu method, and then features are extracted and analysed.

d) Segmentation of optic cup

Arnay et al. [48] proposed a model for retinal fundus images based on ACO and perform optic cup segmentation. They combine the curvature of the vessels with intensity gradient of the optic disc area and will construct the solutions. The agent's capabilities are limited. Agents are capable to find accurate cup segmentation. For testing they have used RIM-ONE dataset.

4.3.4 Cuckoo Search

The Cuckoo search is inspired by the brood parasitism of cuckoo birds. Cuckoo lays their eggs in the nest of other host birds. If a host bird finds that the eggs are not their own, it either throws these alien eggs away or simply abandon its nest to build a new nest elsewhere [49]. Cuckoo search algorithm is a met heuristics optimization algorithm, which is classified into three considerations:

1. Every cuckoo lays approximately one egg at a time and the eggs are exactly set in a nest.

2. The nest having better quality eggs are carried onto the next round.

3. The number of nests is fixed and the quality of nest is static and is not alterable.

The cuckoo search is used in DR models for exudates detection. Srishti et al. [50] design a computational approach based on cuckoo search algorithm for exudates detection using multi-level thresholding; it has been fine-tuned for edge detection. The proposed method starts with initialization of cuckoo with an upper threshold value and lower threshold then selecting a best threshold value via Levy's flight. The threshold value must be less than 0.25. If the value less than maximum than keep threshold values with maximum gradient values otherwise reject. If the maximum iteration obtained then end the process otherwise find best values, keep best threshold values and initialize cuckoo again.

Glaucoma is a main problem for vision loss, which cause increase in fluid pressure in the eye and may damage the optic nerve. So, Raja et al. [51] developed an optimal hyper analytic wavelet transform for glaucoma detection. It is found that by using hybrid GSO- Cuckoo search algorithm they have got an optimal coefficient for transformation process. In this proposed work they give fundus mages as input then pre-process them by using RGB to GRAY scale conversion histogram equalizer. For optimal transformation, author used hyper analytic wavelet transform and GSO-Cuckoo search and give the statistical features to classification modules i.e. ANN and SVM. The methods and salient feature used by the authors for research are shown in Table 4.5.

4.3.5 Bee Colony Optimization

It is a powerful algorithm of artificial intelligence; it is a swarm-based meta-heuristic optimization algorithm inspired by the life cycle of honey bees. There are different honey bee algorithms that have been developed based on the style of building hives, searching under, collecting food, etc. This study will explore the concept of honey bee algorithm. Before explaining the honey bee algorithm it is necessary to understand the lifestyle of honey bees. They look for food in nature by exploring the neighbourhood fields of their hives and collect and accumulate nectar for the future use. To collect food the bees constantly search the region looking for new rubber patches. Once the bee finds food sources, it returns to hive and informs their mates about location, quality and quantity of the available food source [10]. They begin from everything through waggle dance that is move with short quick moment form side to side or ups and downs. In this waggle dance, every movement has different meaning, that is dancing area on hive, number of rounds on

TABLE 4.5   Performance measures of Cuckoo search and bee colony-based models

Author	Method	Salient feature
Srishti et al. [50]	Cuckoo search, PSO, Artificial bee colony	Stationary wavelet transforms
Raja et al. [51]	Cuckoo search, SVM	GSO-Cuckoo, CGD-BPN, Hyper analytic transform
Emary et al. [52]	Bee colony optimization, FCM	ABC-PS multi-objective vessel localization
Hassanien et al. [53]	Artificial bee colony, FCM, Swarm optimization	Compactness fitness function, Bee swarm optimization
Maaneesh and Chaya [54]	Artificial bee colony, FCM	Perform segmentation by assigning each pixel to the cluster
Kavya et al. [55]	Artificial bee colony, FCM, SVM	Fundus camera, vessel segmentation

left side and right side and jumping ups and downs based on these signs will advertise the food location and they encourage the remaining of their colony to follow [11]. After the dance some recruited members follow the scout bee to find the food source to collect more food. This cycle is repeated continuously while the bees are at their hive with accumulated nectar and they explore new areas with a potential food source. In their lifestyle, there are two phases: first is discovering food source and second is collecting food from food sources [12]. This bee colony algorithm is used to make a CAD system for earlier detection of DR. The methods and salient feature used by the authors for research are shown in Table 4.5.

It is important to find accurate segmentation of retinal blood vessels using CAD systems. Emary et al. [52] proposed an automated model for retinal blood vessel segmentation. The model is based on artificial bee colony optimization in collaboration with fuzzy C-means algorithm. Here artificial bee colony algorithm is used to find the cluster center of Fuzzy C-means objective function. This approach is tested on the freely available Drive and stare database. There will be three steps for segmentation of retinal blood vessels: first, to pre-process the data using Band selection and Brightness correction. Second, retinal blood vessel images are given for segmentation then find cluster with ABC using Fuzzy C-means fitness function. Third is post processing which is done by ranking the order filtering, gap filling, non-thin connected component removal methods. Hassanien et al. [53] enlighten us with an approach containing ABC and FCM algorithm in which they focus on the pattern search optimization to enhance the segmentation resulting in a feature called shape description. A fitness function called thinness ratio is used for pattern search optimization. In this they compare to algorithm BSO- and ABC-based approaches in terms of sensitivity, specificity and accuracy.

Maaneesh and Chaya [54] also used ABC and FCM algorithm for their proposed approach. After pre-processing initialize the data and randomly putting bees into target images and generate membership matrix and evaluate function gives to recruit bees for the best site and poor bees for the remaining site select the fittest bee from each site by probably off solution. If iteration equals to MNC, then obtain the optimal centroids and do segmentation by assigning each pixel to the cluster for which the membership value is higher, otherwise replace the solution with a new randomly produced solution by scout bee and construct new population of scout bee. Kavya et al. [55] proposed a system to classify the images through level of damage in blood vessels using support vector machine. Author has used ABC algorithm to improve the accuracy of the system and FCM to assign the values of membership to the pixels.

4.4 CONCLUSION

It is observed that in previous decades diabetes has given rise to number of health issues witnessed universally and increasing day by day. The most common issue caused by diabetes is DR. DR majorly affects human retina and leads to complete vision loss. Few key features of DR are MA, HE, HEM, SE or CWS, and NVD. Traditionally, doctor's manually check the patients and take decisions for the society. It is very complicated to identify DR with complex features. In this context, to fight with the current problem of DR, industries move towards CAD. CAD system enables optimal diagnosis decisions and early DR detection. The automatic DR detection model takes DR images as input to perform various experiments on different models made by different algorithm. Swarm intelligence and EC algorithms play a vital role in dealing with earlier identification of DR. GA, PSO algorithm, ant colony algorithm, bee colony algorithm and cuckoo search algorithms of evolutionary computing and swarm optimization are used to make automatic CAD system for earlier detection of DR. In this chapter, number of CAD system and approaches developed for DR have been studied and assessed on the basis of strength and weakness of the approach. The automatic DR models follow pre-processing, feature extraction, segmentation and classification. Here methods and salient features uses for feature extraction and classification are explored on a large scale.

REFERENCES

[1] Mansour, R. F. (2017). Evolutionary computing enriched computer-aided diagnosis system for diabetic retinopathy: a survey. *IEEE reviews in biomedical engineering*, 10, 334–349.

[2] World Diabetes Foundation, "*A Newsletter from the World Health Organization*," WHO, Geneva, Switzerland, 1998.

[3] Ong, G. L., Ripley, L. G., Newsom, R. S., Cooper, M., & Casswell, A. G. (2004). Screening for sight-threatening diabetic retinopathy: comparison of fundus photography with automated color contrast threshold test. *American journal of ophthalmology*, 137(3), 445–452.

[4] Maher, R. S., Kayte, S. N., Meldhe, S. T., & Dhopeshwarkar, M. (2015). Automated diagnosis non-proliferative diabetic retinopathy in fundus images using support vector machine. *International Journal of Computer Applications, 125*(15).

[5] Mookiah, M. R. K., Acharya, U. R., Chua, C. K., Lim, C. M., Ng, E. Y. K., & Laude, A. (2013). Computer-aided diagnosis of diabetic retinopathy: A review. *Computers in biology and medicine, 43*(12), 2136–2155.

[6] Yun, W. L., Acharya, U. R., Venkatesh, Y. V., Chee, C., Min, L. C., & Ng, E. Y. K. (2008). Identification of different stages of diabetic retinopathy using retinal optical images. *Information sciences, 178*(1), 106–121.

[7] Levels, E. T. D. R. S. (2002). International clinical diabetic retinopathy disease severity scale detailed table. Available Online: www.icoph.org/standards/pdrdetail.html.

[8] Williams, R., Airey, M., Baxter, H., Forrester, J. K. M., Kennedy-Martin, T., & Girach, A. (2004). Epidemiology of diabetic retinopathy and macular oedema: a systematic review. *Eye, 18*(10), 963.

[9] Nayyar, A., Garg, S., Gupta, D., & Khanna, A. (2018). Evolutionary computation: theory and algorithms. In *Advances in Swarm Intelligence for Optimizing Problems in Computer Science* (pp. 1–26). Chapman and Hall/CRC, USA.

[10] Kumar S., Nayyar A., Kumari R. (2019) Arrhenius Artificial Bee Colony Algorithm. In: Bhattacharyya S., Hassanien A., Gupta D., Khanna A., Pan I. (eds) International Conference on Innovative Computing and Communications. Lecture Notes in Networks and Systems, vol 56. Springer, Singapore.

[11] Nayyar A., Puri V., Suseendran G. (2019) Artificial Bee Colony Optimization—Population-Based Meta-Heuristic Swarm Intelligence Technique. In: Balas V., Sharma N., Chakrabarti A. (eds) Data Management, Analytics and Innovation. Advances in Intelligent Systems and Computing, vol 839. Springer, Singapore.

[12] Sharma S., Kumar S., Nayyar A. (2019) Logarithmic Spiral Based Local Search in Artificial Bee Colony Algorithm. In: Duong T., Vo NS. (eds) Industrial Networks and Intelligent Systems. INISCOM 2018. Lecture Notes of the Institute for Computer Sciences, Social Informatics and Telecommunications Engineering, vol 257. Springer, Cham.

[13] Early Treatment Diabetic Retinopathy Study Research Group. (1991). Grading diabetic retinopathy from stereoscopic color fundus photographs—an extension of the modified Airlie House classification: ETDRS report number 10. *Ophthalmology, 98*(5), 786–806.

[14] Alghadyan, A. A. (2011). Diabetic retinopathy–An update. *Saudi Journal of Ophthalmology, 25*(2), 99–111.

[15] McLeod, D. (2005). Why cotton wool spots should not be regarded as retinal nerve fibre layer infarcts. *British Journal of Ophthalmology, 89*(2), 229–237.

[16] Chui, T. Y., Thibos, L. N., Bradley, A., & Burns, S. A. (2009). The mechanisms of vision loss associated with a cotton wool spot. *Vision research*, *49*(23), 2826–2834.

[17] Vallabha, D., Dorairaj, R., Namuduri, K., & Thompson, H. (2004, November). Automated detection and classification of vascular abnormalities in diabetic retinopathy. In *Conference Record of the Thirty-Eighth Asilomar Conference on Signals, Systems and Computers, 2004.* (Vol.2, pp. 1625–1629). IEEE.

[18] Giancardo, L., Meriaudeau, F., Karnowski, T. P., Li, Y., Garg, S., Tobin Jr, K.W., & Chaum, E. (2012). Exudate-based diabetic macular edema detection in fundus images using publicly available datasets. *Medical image analysis*, *16*(1), 216–226.

[19] Frank, R. N. (1991). On the pathogenesis of diabetic retinopathy: a 1990 update. *Ophthalmology*, *98*(5), 586–593.

[20] Osareh, A., Shadgar, B., & Markham, R. (2009). A computational-intelligence-based approach for detection of exudates in diabetic retinopathy images. *IEEE Transactions on Information Technology in Biomedicine*, *13*(4), 535–545.

[21] Rashid, S. (2013). Computerized exudate detection in fundus images using statistical feature based fuzzy c-mean clustering. *International Journal of Computing and digital systems*, *218*(1222), 1–11.

[22] Naluguru. U. Kumar and R. Tirumala, "A cross layer approach for feature extraction with accurate detection through blood vessel segmentation in automatic diabetic retinopathy," Aust. J. Basic Appl. Sci., vol. 9, no. 36, pp. 524–534, Dec. 2015.

[23] Karegowda, A. G., Nasiha, A., Jayaram, M. A., & Manjunath, A. S. (2011). Exudates detection in retinal images using back propagation neural network. *International Journal of Computer Applications*, *25*(3), 25–31.

[24] Ganesan, K., Martis, R. J., Acharya, U. R., Chua, C. K., Min, L. C., Ng, E. Y. K., & Laude, A. (2014). Computer-aided diabetic retinopathy detection using trace transforms on digital fundus images. *Medical & biological engineering & computing*, *52*(8), 663–672.

[25] Nirosha, T., Rao, K. N., & Ratnam, G. S. (2015). Computer aided detection of diabetes retinopathy and analysis through ANFIS and optimtool. *Int. J. Eng. Comput. Sci.*, *4*(9), 14187–14191.

[26] Santos, T., Ribeiro, L., Lobo, C., Bernardes, R., & Serranho, P. (2012, February). Validation of the automatic identification of eyes with diabetic retinopathy by OCT. In *2012 IEEE 2nd Portuguese Meeting in Bioengineering (ENBENG)* (pp. 1–4). IEEE.

[27] Quellec, G., Lamard, M., Josselin, P. M., Cazuguel, G., Cochener, B., & Roux, C. (2008). Optimal wavelet transform for the detection of microaneurysms in retina photographs. *IEEE transactions on medical imaging*, *27*(9), 1230–1241. VC.

[28] Akram, M. U., Tariq, A., Khan, S. A., & Bazar, S. A. (2013, November). Microaneurysm detection for early diagnosis of diabetic retinopathy. In

2013 International Conference on Electronics, Computer and Computation (ICECCO) (pp. 21–24). IEEE.

[29] Lee, N., Laine, A. F., & Smith, R. T. (2007, August). A hybrid segmentation approach for geographic atrophy in fundus auto-fluorescence images for diagnosis of age-related macular degeneration. In *2007 29th Annual International Conference of the IEEE Engineering in Medicine and Biology Society* (pp. 4965–4968). IEEE.

[30] Hung, Y. W., Hsieh, M. Y., Wang, C. L., Yu, S. S., Chan, Y. K., Tsai, M. F., ... & Tung, K. C. (2016). The detections of retinopathy symptoms and tractional retinal detachment. *Advances in Mechanical Engineering, 8*(1), 1687814015624332.

[31] Nayyar, A., & Nguyen, N. G. (2018). Introduction to Swarm Intelligence. *Advances in Swarm Intelligence for Optimizing Problems in Computer Science,* 53–78. Chapman and Hall/CRC, USA.

[32] Nayyar, A., Le, D. N., & Nguyen, N. G. (Eds.). (2018). *Advances in Swarm Intelligence for Optimizing Problems in Computer Science.* CRC Press, USA.

[33] Durbhaka G.K., Selvaraj B., Nayyar A. (2019) Firefly Swarm: Metaheuristic Swarm Intelligence Technique for Mathematical Optimization. In: Balas V., Sharma N., Chakrabarti A. (eds) Data Management, Analytics and Innovation. Advances in Intelligent Systems and Computing, vol 839. Springer, Singapore.

[34] Anitha, J., Vijila, C. K. S., & Hemanth, D. J. (2009). Comparative analysis of genetic algorithm & particle swarm optimization techniques for SOFM based abnormal retinal image classification. *International Journal of Recent Trends in Engineering, 2*(3), 143.

[35] Balakrishnan, U., Venkatachalapathy, K., & S Marimuthu, G. (2015). A hybrid PSO-DEFS based feature selection for the identification of diabetic retinopathy. *Current diabetes reviews, 11*(3), 182–190.

[36] Ravivarma, P., Ramasubramanian, B., Arunmani, G., & Babumohan, B. (2014, May). An efficient system for the detection of exudates in colour fundus images using image processing technique. In *2014 IEEE International Conference on Advanced Communications, Control and Computing Technologies* (pp. 1551–1553). IEEE.

[37] Sreejini, K. S., & Govindan, V. K. (2015). Improved multiscale matched filter for retina vessel segmentation using PSO algorithm. *Egyptian Informatics Journal, 16*(3), 253–260.

[38] Sreejini, K. S., & Govindan, V. K. (2013, August). Automatic grading of severity of diabetic macular edema using color fundus images. In *2013 Third International Conference on Advances in Computing and Communications* (pp. 177–180). IEEE.

[39] Devasia, T., Jacob, P., & Thomas, T. (2015). Automatic Optic Disc Localization and Segmentation using Swarm Intelligence. *World of Computer Science & Information Technology Journal, 5*(6).

[40] Nayyar, A., & Singh, R. (2016, March). Ant colony optimization—computational swarm intelligence technique. In *2016 3rd International conference on*

computing for sustainable global development (INDIACom) (pp. 1493–1499). IEEE.

[41] Bajčeta, M., Sekulić, P., Djukanović, S., Popovic, T., & Popović-Bugarin, V. (2016, November). Retinal blood vessels segmentation using ant colony optimization. In *2016 13th Symposium on Neural Networks and Applications (NEUREL)*(pp. 1–6). IEEE.

[42] Hooshyar, S., & Khayati, R. (2010, May). Retina vessel detection using fuzzy ant colony algorithm. In *2010 Canadian Conference on Computer and Robot Vision* (pp. 239–244). IEEE.

[43] Asad, A. H., El Amry, E., Hassanien, A. E., & Tolba, M. F. (2013, December). New global update mechanism of ant colony system for retinal vessel segmentation. In *13th International Conference on Hybrid Intelligent Systems (HIS 2013)* (pp. 221–227). IEEE.

[44] Asad, A. H., Azar, A. T., Fouad, M. M. M., & Hassanien, A. E. (2013, September). An improved ant colony system for retinal blood vessel segmentation. In *2013 Federated Conference on Computer Science and Information Systems* (pp. 199–205). IEEE.

[45] Pereira, C., Gonçalves, L., & Ferreira, M. (2013). Optic disc detection in color fundus images using ant colony optimization. *Medical & biological engineering & computing, 51*(3), 295–303.

[46] Karthikeyan, T., & Vembandasamy, K. (2014). A refined continuous ant colony optimization based FP-growth association rule technique on type 2 diabetes. *International Review on Computers and Software (IRECOS), 9,* 1476–1483.

[47] Kavitha, G., & Ramakrishnan, S. (2009, December). Identification and analysis of macula in retinal images using Ant Colony Optimization based hybrid method. In *2009 World Congress on Nature & Biologically Inspired Computing (NaBIC)* (pp. 1174–1177). IEEE.

[48] Arnay, R., Fumero, F., & Sigut, J. (2017). Ant colony optimization-based method for optic cup segmentation in retinal images. *Applied Soft Computing, 52,* 409–417.

[49] Gandomi, A. H., Yang, X. S., & Alavi, A. H. (2013). Cuckoo search algorithm: a metaheuristic approach to solve structural optimization problems. *Engineering with computers, 29*(1), 17–35.

[50] Srishti, V. (2014). Technique based on cuckoo's search algorithm for exudates detection in diabetic retinopathy. *Ophthalmol. Res., Int. J., 2*(1), 43–54.

[51] Raja, C., & Gangatharan, N. (2015). Optimal hyper analytic wavelet transform for glaucoma detection in fundal retinal images. *J. Electr. Eng. Technol., 10*(4), 1899–1909.

[52] Emary, E., Zawbaa, H. M., Hassanien, A. E., Schaefer, G., & Azar, A. T. (2014, July). Retinal blood vessel segmentation using bee colony optimisation and pattern search. In *2014 International Joint Conference on Neural Networks (IJCNN)*(pp. 1001–1006). IEEE.

[53] Hassanien, A. E., Emary, E., & Zawbaa, H. M. (2015). Retinal blood vessel localization approach based on bee colony swarm optimization, fuzzy c-means and pattern search. *Journal of Visual Communication and Image Representation, 31,* 186–196.

[54] P. Maaneesh and H. P. Chaya, "Retinal blood vessel segmentation by FCM clustering and artificial bee colony optimization *Int. J. Elect. Electron. Eng. Telecommun.,* 4(3), 21–26.

[55] Kavya, K., Dechamma, M. G., & Kumar, B. S. (2016). Extraction of retinal blood vessel using artificial bee-colony optimization. *Journal of Theoretical and Applied Information Technology, 88(3),* 535–540.

Swarm Intelligence and Evolutionary Algorithms for Heart Disease Diagnosis

Rajalakshmi Krishnamurthi

Department of Computer Science, Jaypee Institute of Information Technology, Noida, India

5.1 INTRODUCTION

Human heart is an organ made of strongest muscles located between the two lungs in the body. The heart is a fist-sized organ within the chest skeleton compartment. The average number of times the human heart beat is approximately 70 times per minute. The left chamber of the heart is responsible to pump the blood out of heart to different organs throughout the body. The pure blood with oxygen and nutrients are carried by the blood vessels known as arteries and capillaries. Similarly, the right chamber of heart collects the impure, deoxygenated blood from various different organs through blood vessels, known as veins. The liver removes the waste products during the blood circulation process. This system is called "cardiovascular system." The human heart is prone to breakdown and damage due to several factors known as cardiovascular diseases (CVD). Primarily, there are five CVDs, namely coronary heart disease (CHD), stroke, hypertension heart diffusion, rheumatic heart disease, and other associated cardiovascular diseases.

Coronary heart disease (CHD): These diseases are caused due to the problems occurring in the blood vessels that supply blood to the heart muscles. The primary factors that lead to CHD are high cholesterol, high blood pressure, sedentary life style, unhealthy diet, smoking, and alcohol and tobacco use.

Rheumatic heart disease (RHD): This disease is caused due to rheumatic fever. Prolonged rheumatic fever damages the heart valves and heart muscles. The streptococcal bacteria are the primary pathogen that causes this disease.

Cardiac arrhythmias (CA): This cardiovascular disease is caused due to abnormality in the heart beat rhythm. The characteristics of arrhythmias are (1) increased heart beat rhythm greater than 100bpm; (2) decrease in the heart beat rhythm less than 60bpm; (3) asynchronous functioning of heart chambers; and (4) irregular rate of heart pumping. The health conditions that result due to cardiac arrhythmias are (1) decrease in the performance of hemodynamics; (2) natural cardiac pacemaker exhibits abnormal pumping rate; (3) blood conduction process interruption due to blockage of blood vessel pathways; and (4) random heart part takes self-alternative responsibility to control pumping rate of blood.

Congenital heart disease: The structure of heart is malformed due to mutation of genetic factors during the gestation period of childbirth. This disease includes hole within the walls of heart, improper valve function, and improper formation of heart chambers. The primary factor of congenital heart disease includes maternal malnutrition during pregnancy, consanguinity between parents, rubella infection, alcohol, etc.

Stroke: The stroke is also known as cerebrovascular disease. The stroke is the disease that is caused due to the disruption of blood circulation to the brain. The causes of disruption are due to blockage in artery (hemorrhage) and damage of blood vessels (ischemic stroke). The external factors that causes stroke are high blood pressure, arrhythmic heart disorder, cholesterol, diabetics, sedentary life style, and aging.

Hypertension heart disease: In case of the hypertension-based heart disease, the blood pressure shoots up to extremely high grade. The working condition of the heart is degraded due to the increase blood pressure and further leads to disordered functioning of heart. The damages caused due to hypertension are heart failure, heart muscle thickening, coronary artery damages, and several other critical conditions.

Other associated heart diseases: Age, diabetic, smoking, virus, pathogens, mastcells, HIV, AIDS, and TB may associate to cause the heart disease termed as associated heart diseases.

According to statistics of WHO (2019), there exists 17% of annual mortality rate due to CHD. This accounts to about one-third of the mortality caused by other diseases across the globe. CHD has evolved as the killer disease in the recent evolutionary world. Further, from the context of evolutionary genetics, impact toward CHD has been explored by researchers in detail. In recent years, CHD are susceptible to be part of the evolutionary genetics according to [1]. In the recent years, there is significant advancement toward CHD and impact from the perspective of evolutionary genetics. The several evolutionary factors that might lead to CHD are hypertension, metabolic syndrome, and dyslipidemia. These factors lead to high blood pressure, weak lipid and glucose metabolism activities, blood vessel coagulation, and heart inflammation and weak energy metabolism activities.

Key contributions of this chapter are:

- Prediction and Classification of Heart Disease Using Machine Learning/Swarm Intelligence

- Diagnosis of Coronary Artery Disease Using the Evolutionary Algorithm

- Predicting Heart Attacks in Patients Using Artificial Intelligence methods

- Swarm Intelligence-Based Optimization Problem for Heart Disease Diagnosis

- Applying Evolutionary Algorithms for Heart Disease Diagnosis

5.2 PREDICTION AND CLASSIFICATION OF HEART DISEASE USING MACHINE LEARNING/SWARM INTELLIGENCE

5.2.1 Decision Support System

In modern age there is huge amount of complexity associated with decision making towards human problems and needs. Hence, the computer-based information system tends to assure solutions to most of decision-making problems with low cost and time is known as decision support system [2–4]. Further, the advancement in the field of computational data mining techniques and artificial intelligence mechanisms has enhanced the process of computational decision support systems. Such systems engage with knowledge databases and derive cognitive inference based on input data are known as "intelligent decision support systems."

5.2.2 Clinical Decision Support System

In this way, clinical decision support systems (CDSS) are well suitable and desired for the healthcare sector. Primarily, the medical sector involves voluminous amount of data and information referring to diversified medical scenarios and conditions. Usually, such huge amount of medical data is stored in dedicated storage bases. This is an added advantage to analyze the data within the dedicated medical domain. The healthcare process involves various phases namely screening of patients, diagnosis of diseases, treatment procedure for patients, and prognosis phases. Each of these phases generates huge data and has medical and health information buried within it [5,6].

The purpose of CDSS is capable enough to identify useful and important hidden patterns, trending effects and structures that left undetectable from the medical data by naive mechanism or humans. The objective of CDSS are (1) to improve the accuracy of various decision process, (2) transparency, (3) interpretability, (4) comprehensiveness, and (5) optimization of the time and cost involved during execution of entire process of decision making.

Accuracy: It targets to discover the precise knowledge from the learning input data.

Interpretability: It targets complexity in healthcare systems that include semantics of medical data and systems.

Transparency: It targets compactness, the level of understanding in terms of explanation and correctness of decision that made using medical records and its attributes.

Comprehensiveness: It targets to provide generalization of knowledge that are generated through various learning processes.

5.2.3 Heart Disease Datasets

In literature, few datasets are used as standard for modeling the CHD diagnosis. For example, Cleveland heart disease dataset, MIT dataset, South African Heart Disease dataset, and Parsian dataset.

Cleveland heart disease data set: This data set provides information over the presence or absence of heart disease in individual patients [7]. For example, the information recorded that is recorded from each patient includes age, gender, blood pressure, blood sugar, cholesterol level and other medical factors. The data set consists of 303 total number of patient records with four types of classifications such as '0' represents absence of heart disease, '1–4' represent various subcategories of heart disease presence. During feature selection, these 4 types of subclass of presence are combined into one; such '0' represents absence of heart disease, while '1' represents presence of heart disease. Originally, the Cleveland heart disease data sets consist of 75 types of features as enlisted for individual patients. However, for data analysis purpose 13 most favourable features are considered in various literature works that exists. These 13 features are age, sex, chest pain, blood pressure under rest, cholesterol, blood sugar under fasting, ECG results under rest, maximum achieved heart rate, angina, old peak, peak slope due to exercise, vessels colour through fluoroscopy techniques, and thalach. In this set of data, the number of case with heart disease constitutes 46%, while remaining 54% constitutes the absence of heart disease cases.

MITBIH database (arrhythmia): Data set consists of Holter estimation value which was monitored at the sample frequency of 30Hz. The twolead measurements are recorded for duration of 30 minutes. The total number of excerpts participate in the study is 48. The observations are made at the Arrhythmia Laboratory of Beth Israel Hospital, Boston. Out of total 48 excerpts, first 23 records are serialized between 100 and 124, with some missing sequence numbers. The next 23 records are 23 records are serialized between 200 and 234. Further, 24 records are without flaws and normal in class, while remaining 21 records exhibits abnormal class of heart diseases.

MITBIH database (Supraventricular): This data set concerns about the arrhythmias in super ventricular and are supplementary to the data set of arrhythmias. The electro cardiogram signals are recorded for the duration of 30 minutes at the sampling frequency of 128 Hz. The two-level recordings are obtained for 78 excerpts.

MITBIH database (Normal Sinus Rhythm Database): The observations recorded in this data base are from arrhythmia laboratory of Beth Israel Hospital located at Boston. In this case, 18 recordings of long-term ECG are performed.

MITBIH database (Long-Term ECG): In this data set, two sets of 7 recordings of one at 14 hours and second at 22 hours are performed.

South African Heart Disease Data Set: The data set of South African Heart Disease records the details of male patients above age of 15 and under age of 64. The Western Cape region of South Africa is considered for study. The primary concern of data set is about presence or absence of heart disease. There are 465 records present in the data set. Two classes are used namely '0' represents presence of heart disease and '1' represents absence of heart diseases. There are 9 attributes associated with this data set namely (i) systolic blood pressure (ii) tobacco use, (iii) low-density lipoprotein cholesterol, (iv) adiposity, (v) history of genetic inheritance, (vi) obesity, (vii) Type A behaviours, (viii) alcohol, and (ix) age. The data set contains 302 cases out 465 total numbers to be presence of heart disease, which amounts 35% cases of negative class. Further, the remaining 160 cases are classified as absence of heart disease.

Parsian Hospital Dataset: The data set of Parsian Hospital, Karaj, Iran consists of heart disease records of 380 patients. The dataset consists of 32.1% of records as male patients and 67.9% of records as female patients. Out of these records, the patients with high symptoms of heart disease are counted to be 55.26%. The various parameters for the patient information include age, gender blood pressure, sugar level in blood, heart rate, smoking and tobacco, cholesterol in blood.

According to [8], the generic framework for heart disease data analysis is carried through four major steps namely data selection, data pre-processing, data modelling and knowledge evaluation.

5.3 PREDICTING HEART ATTACKS IN PATIENTS USING ARTIFICIAL INTELLIGENCE METHODS (FUZZY LOGIC)

In recent years, the computer technology has gained vital role in medical disease diagnosis and treatments. The medical data are growing in terms of volume and veracity. Hence, the conventional methods of patient information gathering are less significant. The complexity and precise diagnosis of medical disease is essential for patient treatment,unlike the regular database where the Boolean logic is adapted to find information to be true or false [9,10]. The data used for medical diagnosis are often ambitious in nature, and hence the conventional Boolean logic is not suitable. In fact, the database management system requires fuzzy logic to handle ambiguous data and to prevent loss of ambiguous information on such databases. Particularly, the loss of ambiguous information may lead to important information that are required for medical diagnosis. Basically, the fuzzy logic-based data base systems provide support for uncertainty, inaccurate and ambiguous information. The principle of fuzzy logic is to solve challenging problems of medical diagnosis, through many valued methods of logics mathematically well-defined through fuzzy set theory. The fuzzy logic was first introduced by Zahed in 1960. The extended version of Boolean logic is the fuzzy logic methods. Accordingly, in fuzzy logic, a fuzzy variable hold any value between 0 and 1 instead of specific binary values (0 and 1). In addition, the fuzzy logic is capable to derive decision in case of inaccurate and ambiguous data inputs.

5.3.1 Fuzzy Logic Approach for Heart Disease Diagnosis

The fuzzy logic approach has been widely adopted for study and diagnosis of heart diseases due to its effectiveness in handling of ambiguous input data. Basically, the heart disease diagnosis through fuzzy logic consists of four stages namely fuzzification, fuzzy rule base, fuzzy inference engine and defuzzification as shown in Figure 5.1.

Fuzzification: This stage involves three substages namely mapping, membership functions, and conversion. First substage is used to mapping various categorical variables into categorical values. Then, the categorical values are mapped into range of numerical values as shown in Table 5.1 below. Second substage is used to define the membership function for both input and output fuzzy variables. Third substage is used to convert the crisp input data into fuzzy data sets based on the corresponding membership functions [11].

Mapping: The two types of data are considered for fuzzification like input data and output data [40-43]. Under input data, the categorical variables are age, blood pressure, blood sugar and blood cholesterol. These categorical input variables are mapped into four categorical

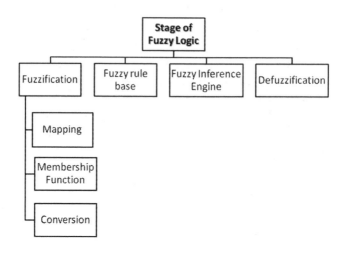

FIGURE 5.1 Stages of fuzzy logic.

TABLE 5.1 Input variables of heart disease diagnosis

Input Variables	Categorical Value	Numerical Range
	Very elderly	> 60
Age	Elder	[45, 65]
	Middle age	[35, 50]
	Adult	[0,38]
Sugar level in blood	High	>110
	Low	<120
	Very high	>160
Systolic blood pressure	High	140–165
	Medium	120–145
	Low	<125
	High	>235
Cholesterol in serum	Medium	190–240
	Low	<125

values namely very elderly, elderly, middle age and adult. Next, these categorical values are mapped to their numerical value range. For example, the *very elderly* categorical value is defined as numerical value greater than 60, the *elder age* is mapped to numerical range between 45 and 65. Similarly, the other input categorical variables, i.e. blood pressure, blood sugar and blood cholesterol are considered. The output data defines the categorical variable namely *result* indicating the presence of disease and it comprises of categorical values namely healthy, moderately healthy, unhealthy with their corresponding numerical range as [0,1.6], [1.5, 2.6] and [2.5,4].

Membership function: In the heart disease diagnosis, the trapezoidal [12] and Gaussian membership functions [13] are commonly used due to efficient result outcomes. In this process, the numerical value defined for various categorical variables are transformed into fuzzy sets based on the membership function.

Trapezoidal membership function is defined using:

$$T(x, a, b, c) = \begin{cases} 0, x \leq a \\ \frac{x-a}{b-a}, a \leq x < b \\ 1, b \leq x < c \\ \frac{d-x}{d-c}, a \leq x < b \\ x, x \geq 0 \end{cases}.$$

Gaussian membership function is defined using two parameters namely mean (μ) and variance (σ^2) as given below equation:

$$G(x, \sigma, \mu) = e^{\frac{-(x-c)^2}{2\sigma^2}}$$

5.3.2 Fuzzy Rule Base

In the fuzzy logic system, fuzzy rules are constructed to generate knowledge based and get control on the appropriate output variable. The structure of fuzzy rule consists of IF-THEN semantics, that includes first a condition has to be satisfied, then as an output, conclusion is derived. These rules are constructed based on the various input and output parameters of the data sets. Thus, fuzzy rule base play vital role in any fuzzy inference system. However, the quality of the fuzzy rule base has greater impact on the quality of the output generation. Sample of fuzzy rule base is given in Table 5.2.

TABLE 5.2   Sample fuzzy rule base for heart disease diagnosis

Rule #1 IF *age* is *young* AND *blood pressure* is *low* AND *cholesterol* is *low* AND *blood sugar* is *low* **THEN** *result* is *absence*

Rule#2 IF *age* is *middle-aged* AND *blood pressure* is *medium* AND *cholesterol* is *high* AND *blood sugar* is *high* **THEN** *result* is *presence*

5.3.3 Fuzzy Inference Engine

Fuzzy inference involves process of reasoning that performs mapping of specific input data to an appropriate output based on fuzzy logic [8]. Particularly, the fuzzy rule base is used to conduct evaluation of the interference. Generally, the Mamdani Model is used for the fuzzy inference. Finally, the aggregation operation is performed to consolidate all independent fuzzy based outputs into a single set of fuzzy output. For aggregation operation, the AND operator is used.

5.3.4 Defuzzification

The defuzzification involves the process of converting aggregated output of fuzzy into a corresponding numerical output value. Generally, the common method of defuzzification is through centre of gravity (COG), which is defined by equation as given below:

$$x^* = \frac{\int (\alpha_x^* t)dt}{\int \alpha_x dt}$$

Gorzalczany and Rudzinski [12] discussed the decision support system for diagnosing heart diseases based on the fuzzy logic concept. The authors discussed the multi objective optimization using several significant techniques such as NSGA II, SPEA, and MOEOA. The fuzzy logic-based learning machine consists of four steps. First step is to learn about data that involves both input and output of the learning samples. Second step is creating knowledge base that consists of logic rule base and the data information base. The logic rule base is of linguistic nature. During genetic algorithm (GA)-based learning process, these fuzzy logic rules are optimized. For this purpose, the original data, cross over parameter, and mutation parameter for GAs are appropriately defined. Thirdly, the representation of various input attributes and labels for classification are defined. In the next step, the fuzzy logic-based inference engine is defined. Finally, in the last step, multi objective optimization based on the accuracy measure and the interpretability is performed. For accuracy, the maximization of the accuracy factor is considered as the objective function. Similarly, in case of interpretability, the objective function is defined as the maximization process. For solving this multiple objective function Multi object Evolutionally Optimization algorithm (MO-EOA) is used.

5.4 PREDICTING HEART DISEASE USING GENETIC ALGORITHMS

GAs are based on the Darwin's theory of genetic evolution and natural selection. In each generation, the population represents the solution search space. Each individual in the population is represented through chromosome. Each chromosome consists of genes of fixed size. Each gene within an individual chromosome is encoded as random binary value. The GA has three fundamental functions namely Evaluation, Selection, and Reproduction along with appropriate training model [14].

Evaluation: During this process the training data set is evaluated for the assigned with weight vectors. And then the effectiveness of the weights assigned is estimated. This estimation is utilized during selection process. The objective of the evaluation function is programmer specific. The generalized format for evaluation function of Nsize of training data set is given below.

$$E(\gamma) = \sum_{k=1}^{N} \gamma_i$$

$$\gamma_i = \begin{cases} 0, & s^i \text{ is incorrect classification} \\ f(\omega^i), & \text{otherwise} \end{cases}$$

where s^i the training data where $f(s)$ is function monotonic decreasing order.

Selection: During process, the population suitable for breeding is performed. The probability-based selection of the weight vector ω^i is carried out based on the fitness parameter v^i. The ranking of the weight vector is estimated for M number of weight vectors using the formula given below for a particular population.

$$P(\omega^i) = \frac{2v^i}{M(M+1)}$$

Reproduction: The reproduction process in GA consists of three parameters namely crossover, cloning and mutation. The primary objective of these parameters is to fine tune the required changes to reproduce next decedents of current population [14]. During crossover operation, the two parent weight vectors are crossed over at random points to generate new decedents. During mutation operation, the single weight vector is mutated at random points to generate new mutated weight vectors. In cloning operation, one weight vector of an individual is replicated to produce exactly same weight vector as new decedent.

These above described three function of GA are repeated over several iterations until the optimal solution is obtained for the given objective function. Ahkoondi and Hoseeini [13] and Samuel et al. [15] discussed the prognosis of Heart disease using fuzzy logic expert system, while tuning of membership function through GA. In this authors, proposed the Mamdani model and optimization of the defined problem is carried out using hybridization of fuzzy logic and GA. Authors exhibited that accuracy of the proposed hybrid fuzzy-GA method as 92.37%. The model considered two performance factors namely accuracy and interpretability for the prognosis mechanism of heart disease. The proposed mechanism involved steps such as designing of Fuzzy Inference System (FIS). Next, to identify the necessary parameters to performance optimization using GA, the chromosome was then formatted. The objective function and the tuning parameters were formulated. Then, the several GA parameters were appropriately set. Next, the individuals were populated and reproduced using mechanism such as crossover and mutation. Finally, the Fuzzy expert system was executed based on optimization through GA parameters. The training data set was obtained from Parsian Hospital, Karaj, Iran. There were records of 380 patients, with 32.1% of male patients. The high-risk patients accounted for 55.26%. The different features involved in the data set were Sex, age, blood pressure, heart rate, smoking habit, cholesterol level and sugar levels. KaanUyar [16] issued the heart disease diagnosis based on GA and recurrent fuzzy neural network (RFNN). Polat et al. [17] and Polat et al. [18] discussed how data pre-processing through fuzzy logic used to monitor immune system monitoring and heart disease diagnosis. Anooj [19] proposed the implementation of weighted attributes for fuzzy rule-based medical diagnosis support system. Gorzalczany and Rudzinski [12] discussed the diagnosis heart disease based on the fuzzy systems as the objective problem. The first objective is to maximize the interpretability. In which the fuzzy logic is used to reduce the number of rules and thus reduce the complexity. The second objective is to maximize the accuracy such the number of correct decisions are improved. To solve the multiple objective and to derive the optimal solution GA is used. Al-Milli [20] discussed the backpropagation based neural network for CHD.

5.5 SWARM INTELLIGENCE BASED OPTIMIZATION PROBLEM FOR HEART DISEASE DIAGNOSIS

5.5.1 Ant Colony Optimization

ACO optimization is motivated based on the life system of ant colony behaviour. Basically, concept of ACO is the foraging activity of these ants, to find the shortest path from its nest to the target food [21–23]. The foraging process is performed by ant using chemical deposit known as *Pheromone*, such that every ant that passes through the pheromone reaches their target food optimally. In addition to the pheromone deposited by other ants on the path, each ant utilizes self-instinct based on smell of food know as *heuristics* to decide the best path to target food. Once, the self-determined path is decided, the ant confirms the self-decision path by depositing pheromone of its own, thus adding dense to the existing pheromone path. As the result of this learning process, based on individual ant behaviour, the shortest path from the nest to food and then back to nest is identified. It was observed that even if there exists several possible equal paths between nest and food, the pheromone path is denser on particular shortest path. Further, as time passes on, the shortest path is reinforced through pheromone deposits. Ant colony optimization (ACO) mechanism is based on this pheromone trailing process of ant life system. In ACO, to achieve the optimized solution of shortest path, the quantity of pheromone deposit is considered as main parameter. It is being noted that, the pheromone deposit is inverse proportional to the path length between source and the destination. The objective of the ACO algorithm is defined as to find the shortest path in a given graph G (V, E), with V vertices and E edges.

$$
P_{a \to b}^{n} = \begin{cases} \dfrac{\rho_{a \to b}^{\gamma} h_{a \to b}^{\beta}}{\sum_{s \in path(t,I)} \rho_{a \to s}^{\gamma} h_{a \to s}^{\beta}}, \forall j \in path(t, I) \\ 0, otherwise \end{cases}
$$

where $P_{a \to b}^{n}$ represents the probability such that ant n will choose the path (V_a, V_b) from set of vertices V. The parameter $\rho_{a \to b}^{\gamma}$ represents the pheromone characteristics and the parameter $h_{a \to b}^{\beta}$ represents the heuristic information at time t. The $path(t, I)$ represents the set of all possible paths while satisfying various constraints of the objective function.

5.5.2 Particle Swarm Optimization

The swarm behaviour of bird flocks, fish school, and insects has inspired to develop the set of optimization algorithms known as particle swarm optimization (PSO) [24]. In the scenario of bird flock, the birds are intended to find food without any prior knowledge of exact food location [10]. Based on the institution developed by each bird over the course of time is utilized to make decision to find exact nutriments for the entire bird flock. The advantage of this approach is that every individual of the school participate in decision making and there is no collision among individuals during distributed search for nutriments. In case of PSO, the swarm is considered to be particles that are flying within the search space in order to find the feasible solution. The velocity of each particle is defined by their current best position in the search space and the distance to reach the global best position. The various information handled by each particle is namely current position (C_i), current velocity (V_i), individual best know position (B_i), global best know position (G_i).

The objective function f is defined as to find the best possible position of all the individual particles and given in below equation ().

$$
B_i(t + 1) = \begin{cases} B_i(t), & iff(C_i(t + 1)) \geq f(B_i(t)) \\ C_i(t + 1), & iff(C_i(t + 1)) < f(B_i(t)) \end{cases}
$$

Then the function for global best position of individual particles are given by equation

$$
G(t) = min\{f(B_0(t)), f(B_1(t)), f(B_2(t)), \dots, f(B_n(t))\}
$$

The velocity and current position are updated during each iteration in PSO algorithm, based on two parameters namely weight 'w', acceleration constant 'a' and random value 'r'. The function for updating of velocity and current position as given below equation () & ()

$$V_i(t+1) = w^* V_i(t) + a_1 r_1(t)(B_i(t) - C_i(t) + a_2 r_2(t)(B_i(t) - C_i(t)$$
$$C_i(t+1) = C_i(t) + V_i(t+1)$$

The termination condition for PSO algorithm is the convergence of velocity almost to zero. In addition to the objective function, a fitness function is defined to determine the optimal solution for the given problem.

Hedeshi and Abadeh [25], Reddy and Khare [26] and Sagir and Sathsivam [27], discussed a diagnosis system for heart disease based on hybridization of two powerful techniques. The fuzzy inference system is combined with the PSO algorithm. The data set of UCI Cleveland and Hungarian were considered for modelling the heart disease diagnosis. The output was angiography-based status, to classify the presence of disease at various stages. The experimentation results depicted that 93.27% as achieved accuracy while performing the classification of heart disease. Hedeshi and Abadeh [25] discussed the hybridized mechanism for heart disease prediction. In this mechanism the Rough Set was combined with PSO algorithm. The clinical parameters based on UCI machine learning data set repository were considered for modelling the problem. The classification of heart disease output comprised of 3 major classes. The experimentation output depicted that 95.25% accuracy was achieved in prediction of heart diseases. Dilmac and Korurek [28] proposed the extended version of Artificial Bee Colony algorithm for the classification of heart rate. The input parameters were based on heart beat obtained through ECG monitoring. The system produced 7 different relevant clusters that corresponded to different heart diseases. The data set were based on MITBIH database. The experimentation result achieved sensitivity of 99.46%, specificity of 99.37% and positive productivity of 99.94%. Turabieh [29] discussed the combined mechanism of ANN and Gray Wolf Optimization algorithm for heart disease diagnosis. Figure 5.2 depicts the generic flow diagram for PSO-based data analysis in heart disease diagnosis process.

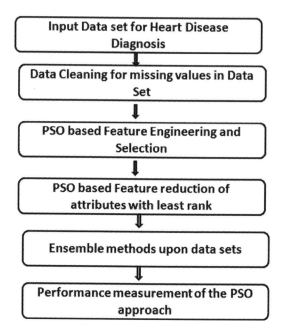

FIGURE 5.2   Flow diagram for particle swarm optimization based data analysis of heart disease diagnosis.

5.6 HEART DISEASE PREDICTION USING DATA MINING TECHNIQUES

There are four major data mining techniques incorporated in heart disease prediction, i.e. association rule, classification, clustering and prediction [30].

Association Rules: The objective in association rule-based mechanism is to obtain a hidden pattern between two different elements during each instance of their transactions. In case of predicting heart disease, the association rule is used to explain, analyze and classify the various parameters recorded for each patient. Then forecast the heart disease based on the risk factor derived using various parameters [31].

Classification: The objective of classification mechanism is to map each element that belongs to a particular input data group into one of the predefined data group. Some of the popular techniques under classification are statistical methods, decision tress, neural network and linear program-ming [27].

Clustering: The objective of clustering is to group elements with similar property into a specific cluster. In case of heart disease forecasting, this method is useful by grouping patients with identical risk factors corre-lated to any explicit heart problem [4].

Prediction: The objective of prediction is to derive the relationship between each dependent element and the independent elements of the data sets. In case of heart disease prediction, each dependent and inde-pendent elements of input data set is analyzed to obtain the relationship.

In literature, the commonly tools used for data mining in heart disease diagnosis are Weka [32,33], MATLAB [24], TANAGRA [34], Statistical Analysis System (SAS) software [11]. The data mining techni-ques are Naive Bayes, Neural Networks, Decision Trees [35], Fuzzy logic [36], and Multilayer Perceptrons [29]. Yang et al. [8] discussed the diagnosis of vavular malfunction-based heart disease using neural net-work techniques. The authors used SAS software for experimentation and achieved maximum accuracy as 97.4%. Also, they showed 89.01% accuracy for diagnosis of comprehensive heart diseases. Bhatla and Jyoti [34]dis-cussed different data mining techniques for heart diseases diagnosis, namely Navie Bayes, Neural Network and Decision Tree. The various tools like Weka, net platform, TANGRA were used. It was noted that accuracy of 99% was achieved using Weka tool and Naive Bayes mechan-ism. Whereas minimum of 45% accuracy was achieved using decision tree under TANGRA software. Alizadehsami et al. [37] studied various data mining techniques like C4.5, multilayer perceptron, and neural network using Weka tool. Under this, the accuracy of 100% was achieved for prediction of heart disease as part of health care decision support system. Taneja [32] discussed J48 and Naive Bayes algorithms for Heart disease diagnosis using Weka tool. The authors has achieved maximum of 95.54% accuracy under various experimentation scenarios.

In case of CHD, the input data consists of three significant attributes inorder to facilitate the prediction process. These attributes are age, sex and symptom intensity. The output attribute for prediction was a single value that represents the presence of disease in the particular patient. In case of coronary artery diseases (CAD), the transformation parameters correspond to heart blood vessels. The level of narrowing in the blood vessel indicates the health condition of artery. The blood vessels presenting the artery disease are left anterior descending (LAD) artery, right coronary artery (RCA), left circumflex (LCX) artery and left main (LM) coronary artery. The evaluation points for measuring the CAD based on LCX, RCA and LAD artery laid between 50% and 70%. In cardiovascular clinical observation, an artery narrowing evaluation value below 50% represents the health artery. The clinical value above 50% represents the patient with borderline artery disease. Finally, the clinical evaluation value 70% and above represents patient suffering from significant heart disease. The fourth critical artery is the LM blood vessel. The clinical threshold point for LM artery is between 30% and 50%. The reason is that LM contributes toward heart disease. The more the blockage of LM artery, the probability of heart disease is higher level than other three arteries. Dangare and Apte. [33] provided an overview of different data mining techniques for heart disease prediction. The decision tree algorithms have further variants namely C4.5, Iterative Dichotomized 3 (ID3) and Classification and Regression Tree (CART). In this chapter, the different heart disease diagnosis through various evaluation techniques were analyzed and compared. The main aim was to develop a systematic prototype for knowledge generation based on the patient medical records to diagnosis heart disease. For this purpose, hybridization of GA was incorporated. The authors purport that this prototype is significant to the medical practitioners to make correct decision on heart disease and hence facilitate toprovide timely recovery treatments for the patients. Bouktif [21] and Jabbar et al.[38] performed evaluative study on state-of-the-art work in research community towards diagnosis and prediction methods for heart diseases. The data mining techniques like Naive Bayes, K-nearest Neighbour Classification, Support Vector Machine, and Artificial Neural Network were considered for the purpose. Nguyen et al. [41], SVM exhibited overall performance and highly promising in the prediction of CHD. In case of CVD diagnosis, the decision tree-based feature reduction exhibited significant classification.

5.7 PERFORMANCE METRICS

The performance of various diagnosis techniques that are used for heart disease diagnosis are measured through seven metrics namely

Root Mean Square Error (RMSE), Accuracy, Sensitivity, Specificity, Probability of the misclassification error (PME), F-score, Precision [39]. The various test cases are measure based on four factors namely True Negative (TN), False Negative (FN), True Positive (TP), and False Positive (FP) as depicted in the Table 5.3 below. Further, Table 5.4 below provides summary of various works carried out in heart disease

These tests are carried out on training data set, testing data set and performance of the heart disease decision support system in whole. The mainly three parameters are used in estimating these metrics namely actual input value (I), output (O) and diagnosis transaction (t).

TABLE 5.3   Test cases for performance analysis of heart disease diagnosis

True Negative	T_{Neg}	Clinical test result shows patient without heart disease and has no heart disease in actual.
False Negative	F_{Neg}	Clinical test result shows patient without heart disease and has heart disease in actual.
True Positive	T_{Pos}	Clinical test result shows patient heart disease and has heart disease in actual.
False Positive	F_{Pos}	Clinical test result shows patient heart disease and has no heart disease in actual.

TABLE 5.4   Comparison of various works carried out in heart disease

Heart Disease Methodology	Author, Year	Technique	Accuracy
Heart Disease Prediction	Shathesh (2016)	Particle Swarm Optimization, Rough set	95.25%
	Nabeel (2013)	Propagation neural network	92%
	Santhanam (2015)	Fuzzy inference system, GA	86%
	Long (2015)	Rough set, Fuzzy logic	86%
Heart Disease Classification	Dilmac (2015)	Artificial bee colony algorithm	99.94%
	Nguyen (2015)	Fuzzy and Genetic Algorithm	95.59%
	Jabbar (2013)	KNN, Genetic Algorithm	95.73%
	Rana (2016)	Fuzzy expert systems, Mamdani Model	85.52%
Heart Disease Diagnosis	Debabrata (2012)	Fuzzy logic System	83.85%
	Sanz (2011)	Genetic Algorithm and Fuzzy Expert Systems	74%

Root Mean Square Error (RMSE) is the standard deviation of the errors that are predicted as residuals (prediction errors). Residuals provide the measure of distance between regression line and sample data points.

$$RMSE = \sqrt{\frac{1}{N} \sum_{t=1}^{N} (I_t - O_t)^2}$$

Accuracy is defined as the ration between total sums of truly classified heart disease samples to the total number of heart disease samples.

$$Accuracy = \frac{T_{Pos} + T_{Neg}}{T_{Pos} + T_{Neg} + F_{Pos} + F_{Neg}}$$

Sensitive is defined as the ratio between the true positive heart disease samples to the sum of true positive and false negative heart disease samples.

$$Sensitivity = \frac{T_{Pos}}{T_{Pos} + F_{Neg}}$$

Specificity is defined as the ratio between the true negative heart disease samples to the sum of true negative and false positive heart disease samples.

$$Specificity = \frac{T_{Neg}}{T_{Neg} + F_{Pos}}$$

PME is defined as the ration between total sums of falsely classified heart disease samples to the total number of heart disease samples.

$$PME = \frac{F_{Pos} + F_{Neg}}{T_{Pos} + T_{Neg} + F_{Pos} + F_{Neg}}$$

Precision is defined as the ratio between the true positive heart disease samples to the sum of true positive and false positive heart disease samples.

$$Precision = \frac{T_{Pos}}{T_{Pos} + F_{Pos}}$$

F Score is defined as the twice the ratio between product of recall and precision factors to the sum of recall and precision factors.

$$F - Score = 2^* \left(\frac{Recall * Precision}{Recall + Precision} \right)$$

5.8 CONCLUSION

In this chapter, the heart disease diagnosis through various mechanisms was discussed. The overview of different types of heart disease such as CHD, CAD, CVD and associated heart diseases and the prevailing statistics of heart disease as per WHO were elaborated. The chapter further discussed the types of data based that were available for research community, data set details also presented. In context of prediction and Classification of Heart Disease, the vital role-played by machine learning and swarm intelligence were discussed. The Fuzzy inference systems, GAs were discussed in details for heart disease diagnosis. Similarly, the swarm intelligence as such PSO and ACO were discussed. Various performance metrics were also detailed in this chapter. Finally, the comparisons of various results obtained by different authors that exist for heart disease diagnosis were presented.

REFERENCES

[1] Kim, J. K., Lee, J. S., Park, D. K., Lim, Y. S., & Lee, Y. H. (2014). Adaptive mining prediction model for content recommendation to coronary heart disease patients. *Cluster Computing*, 17(3):881–891.

[2] Çiftçi, F. B., & Incekara, H. (2011). Web based medical decision support system application of coronary heart disease diagnosis with Boolean functions minimization method. *Expert Systems with Applications*, 38:14037–14043.

[3] Pal, D., Mandana, K.M., Pal, S., Sarkar, D., & Chakraborty, C. (2012). Fuzzy expert system approach for coronary artery disease screening using clinical parameters. *Knowledge-Based Systems*, 36:162–174.

[4] Shaoa, Y. E., Houa, C. D., & Chiuba, C. C. (2014). Hybrid intelligent modeling schemes for heart disease classification. *Applied Soft Computing*, 14:47–52.

[5] Pramanik, P. K. D., Pareek, G., & Nayyar, A. (2019). Security and privacy in remote healthcare: issues, solutions, and standards. Editor(s): Hemanth D. Jude, Valentina Emilia Balas, In *Telemedicine Technologies*. Academic Press.

[6] Pramanik, P. K. D., Nayyar, A., & Pareek, G. (2019). WBAN: driving e-healthcare beyond telemedicine to remote health monitoring: architecture and protocols. Editor(s): Hemanth D. Jude, Valentina Emilia Balas, In *Telemedicine Technologies* (pp. 89–119). Academic Press.

[7] Bache, K., & Lichman, M. (2013). UCI Machine Learning Repository [http://archive.ics.uci.edu/ml]. University of California, School of Information and Computer Science, Irvine, CA.

[8] Yang, J. G., Kim, J. K., Kang, U. G., & Lee, Y. H. (2014, August). Coronary heart disease optimization system on adaptive-network-based fuzzy inference system and linear discriminant analysis (ANFIS-LDA). *Personal and Ubiquitous Computing*, 18(6):1351–1362.

[9] M. Alsalamah, S. Amin and J. Halloran, "Diagnosis of heart disease by using a radial basis function network classification technique on patients' medical records," 2014 IEEE MTT-S International Microwave Workshop Series on RF and Wireless Technologies for Biomedical and Healthcare Applications (IMWS-Bio2014), London, 2014, pp. 1–4. doi: 10.1109/IMWS-BIO.2014.7032401 .

[10] Paul, A. K., Shill, P. C., Rabin, M. R. I., Kundu, A., & Akhand, M. A. H., 2015. Fuzzy membership function generation using DMS-PSO for the diagnosis of heart disease. In *2015 18th International Conference on Computer and Information Technology (ICCIT)* (pp. 456–461). Dhaka.

[11] Shamsollahi, M., badiee, A., & Ghazan- Fari, M. (2018). Using combined descriptive and predictive methods of data mining for coronary artery disease prediction: a case study approach. *Journal of AI and Data Mining.* v7(1), 47–58.

[12] Gorzałczany, M. B., & Rudzinski, F. (2017). Heart-disease diagnosis decision support employing fuzzy systems with genetically optimized accuracy-interpretability trade-off. In *2017 IEEE Symposium Series on Computational Intelligence (SSCI)* (pp. 1–8). IEEE. doi:10.1109/ssci.2017.8280848

[13] Akhoondi, R., & Hosseini, R. (2016). A fuzzy expert system for prognosis of the risk of development of heart disease. *Journal of Advances in Computer Research*, 7(2):101–114.

[14] Sanz, J., Pagola, M., Bustince, H., Bru-gos, A., Fernandez, A., & Herrera, F. (2011). A case study on medical diagnosis of cardiovascular diseases using a Genetic Algorithm for Tuning Fuzzy Rule-Based Classification Systems with Interval-Valued Fuzzy Sets. In *2011 IEEE Symposium on Advances in Type-2 Fuzzy Logic Systems (T2FUZZ)* (pp. 9–15).

[15] Samuel, O. W., Asogbon, G. M., Sangaiah, A. K., Fang, P., & Li, G. (2017). An integrated decision support system based on ANN and Fuzzy_AHP for heart failure risk prediction. *Expert Systems With Applications*, 68:163–172.

[16] KaanUyar, A. I. (2017). Diagnosis of heart disease using genetic algorithm based trained recurrent fuzzy neural networks. *Procedia Computer Science*, 120, 588–593.

[17] Polat, K., Güneş, S., & Sülayman, T. (2006, November). Diagnosis of heart disease using artificial immune recognition system and fuzzy weighted pre-processing. *Pattern Recognition*, 39(11):2186–2193.

[18] Polat, K., Güneş, S., & Tosun, S. (2006). Diagnosis of heart disease using artificial immune recognition system and fuzzy weighted pre-processing. *Pattern Recognition*, 39:2186–2193.

[19] Anooj, P. K., 2013. Implementing decision tree fuzzy rules in clinical decision support system after comparing with fuzzy based and neural network based systems. In *2013 International Conference on IT Convergence and Security (ICITCS)* (pp. 1–6).

[20] Al-Milli, N. (2013). Backpropagation neural net-work for prediction of heart disease. *Journal of Theoretical and Applied Information Technology*, 56(1):131–135.

[21] Bouktif, S., Hanna, E. M., Zaki, N., & Abu Khousa, E. (2014). Ant colony optimization algorithm for interpretable Bayesian classifiers combination: application to medical predictions. *Plos One*, 9(2): e86456, 12.

[22] Nayyar, A., & Singh, R. (2016, March). Ant colony optimization— computational swarm intelligence technique. In *2016 3rd International Conference on Computing for Sustainable Global Development (INDIACom)* (pp. 1493–1499). IEEE.

[23] Nayyar, A., & Singh, R. (2017). Simulation and performance comparison of ant colony optimization (ACO) routing protocol with AODV, DSDV, DSR routing protocols of wireless sensor networks using NS-2 simulator. *American Journal of Intelligent Systems*, 7(1):19–30.

[24] Muthukaruppan, S., & Er, M. J. (2012). A hybrid particle swarm optimization based fuzzy expert system for the diagnosis of coronary artery disease. *Expert Systems with Applications*, 39(14):11657–11665.

[25] Hedeshi, N. G., & Abadeh, M. S. (2014). Coronary artery disease detection using a fuzzy-boosting PSO approach. *Computational Intelligence and Neuroscience*, Article ID 783734, 12, 2014.

[26] Reddy, G. T., & Khare, N. (2017). An efficient system for heart disease prediction using hybrid OFBAT with rule-based fuzzy logic model. *Journal of Circuits, Systems, and Computers*, 26(4), 1750061.

[27] Sagir, A. M., & Sathasivam, S. (2017). A novel adaptive neuro fuzzy inference system based classification model for heart disease prediction. *Pertanika Journal of Science & Technology*, 25(1):43–56.

[28] Dilmac, S., & Korurek, M. (2015). ECG heart beat classification method based on modified ABC algorithm. *Applied Soft Computing*, 36:641–655.

[29] Turabieh, H. (2016). A hybrid ANN-GWO algorithm for prediction of heart disease. *American Journal of Operations Research*, 6(2):136–146.

[30] Amiri, A. M., & Armano, G., 2013. Early diagnosis of heart disease using classification and regression trees. In *The 2013 International Joint Conference on Neural Networks (IJCNN)* (pp. 1–4). Dallas, TX.

[31] Nahar, J., Imam, T., Tickle, K. S., & Chen, Y.-P.-P. (2013b). Association rule mining to detect factors which contribute to heart disease in males and females. *Expert Systems with Applications*, 40:1086–1093.

[32] Taneja, A. (2013). Heart disease prediction system using data mining techniques. *Oriental Journal Of Computer Science &Technology*, 6(4), 457–466.

[33] Dangare, C., & Apte, S. (2012, October-December). A data mining approach for prediction of heart disease using neural networks (November 14, 2012). *International Journal of Computer Engineering and Technology (IJCET)*, 3(3), 30–40.

[34] Bhatla, N., & Jyoti, K. (2012). A novel approach for heart disease diagnosis using data mining and fuzzy logic.

[35] Jabbar, M. A., Deekshatulu, B. L., & Chndra, P., 2014. Alternating decision trees for early diagnosis of heart disease. In *Proceedings of International Conference on Circuits, Communication, Control and Computing (I4C 2014)* (pp. 322–328). MSRIT, Bangalore, India.

[36] Hussain, A., Wenbi, R., Xiaosong, Z., Hongyang, W., & Da Silva, A. L. (2016). Personal home healthcare system for the cardiac patient of smart city using fuzzy logic. *Journal of Advances in Information Technology*, 7(1), 58–64.

[37] Alizadehsani, R., Habibi, J., Alizadeh Sani, Z., Mashayekhi, H., Boghrati, R., Ghandeharioun, A., Khozeimeh, F., & Alizadeh-Sani, F. (2013, August). Diagnosing coronary artery disease via data mining algorithms by considering laboratory and echocardiography features. *Research in Cardiovascular Medicine*, 2(3):133–139. Epub 2013 Jul 31.

[38] Akhil Jabbar, M., Deekshatulu, B. L., & Priti, C. (2013). Classification of heart disease using K- nearest neighbor and genetic algorithm. *Procedia Technology*, 10:85–94.

[39] Krishnaiah, V., Narsimha, G., & Chandra, N. S. (2016). Heart disease prediction system using data mining techniques and intelligent fuzzy approach: a review. *Heart Disease*, 136(2), 43–51.

[40] Cong Long, N., Meesad, P., & Her-wig, U. (2015). A highly accurate firefly based algorithm for heart disease prediction. *Expert Systems with Applications*, 42(21):8221–8231.

[41] Nguyen, T., Khosravi, A., Creighton, D., & Nahavandi, S. (2015). Medical data classification using interval type-2 fuzzy logic system and wavelets. *Applied Soft Computing*, 30:812–822.

[42] Shathesh, S., & Durairaj, M. (2016). An intelligent hybrid mechanism to predict the risk of cardio vascular disease. *Indian Journal of Science and Technology*, 9(4):137–146.

[43] Nguyen, T., Khosravi, A., Creighton, D., & Nahavandi, S. (2015). Classification of healthcare data using genetic fuzzy logic system and wavelets. *Expert Systems with Applications*, 42(4):2184–2197.

Swarm Intelligence and Evolutionary Algorithms for Drug Design and Development

Bandana Mahapatra

School of Mechnatronics, Symbiosis Skills and Open University, Pune, India

6.1 INTRODUCTION

Drug design, also termed as the general drug design, is a research methodology of finding new medications based upon the knowledge of the biology targets [1]. The drugs or medications are nothing but the organic small molecules that activate or inhibit the function of a biomolecule-like protein which results in a therapeutic benefit to the patient [2,3]. The procedure of drug design is about designing the molecules which are complementary in both the shape and charge to the bimolecular target which they would interact as well as bind with. The drug design process majorly, but not necessarily, depends upon the computer modelling techniques [4]. This style of modelling is otherwise known as computer-aided drug design. On the other hand, the drug designing process lying over the knowledge of three-dimensional structure of the biomolecular target is known as the "structure-based drug design" [5].

Few vital classes of the computational methods have improved the affinity, selectivity and stability. Small molecules, biopharmaceuticals which include peptides, therapeutics antibodies, etc., have together contributed in developing the protein-based therapeutics.

117

It can be said that, drug designing to certain extent is a misnomer [6]. A more accurate term is ligand design, which describes the design of a molecule that binds tightly to the target. Though the designing techniques for predicting the binding affinity are quite successful, there are many varied properties, e.g. bio-availability, metabolic half-life, side effects, etc., which need optimization as primary factor prior to ligand becoming safe and efficacious drug [7]. These characteristics are generally tough to predict with the rational design technique. Due to the high attrition rates, specifically during the chemical phases of the drug development, more attention is being focused at the early stages of drug designing process like selecting the candidate drugs whose psychochemical properties can be predicted. These mentioned stages may result in few complicacies during development process making improved as well as marketed drug more popular and apt for usage [6,8].

Currently, in vitro experiments complemented with the computational methods have been widely used in the process of early drug discovery in order to select compounds with more favorable ADME (absorption, distribution, metabolism and excretion) as well as the toxicology profiles.

In the year 1949, while nitrogen mustard alkylating agent mechloretha-mine was launched in the market, the average life expectancy of the cancer victims worldwide was 46.8 years [9,10]. By 2015, almost 160 kinds of anticancer drugs were available in the market raising the average life expectancy to 71.4 years as reported by World Health Statistics, 2017. The rise in death rates due to diseases like cancer can be attributed to the demographic changes. Currently, cancer may be considered as the second largest death causing disease according to World Health Statistics, 2017. This triggers the consistent efforts put by the drug developers in order to design most demanded, new antineoplastic agents against other anticancer drugs available in the market [10].

The increase in the number of anticancer agents available in the market after 1980s can be accounted to two novel oncological drugs every year. These numbers back significantly the amount of money invested by pharmaceutical companies in cancer research due to the result of constant growth of antineoplastic agents worldwide. The rise in demand has given way to the increase in sales in this therapeutic area, e.g. paclitaxel, a popular microtubule stabilizer, the first anti-cancer drug reached the sales of $1 billion during late 1990s. Today, the top 10 antineoplastic drugs have reached the sales target of about $1 billion [11,12].

The sales of drugs have notably risen along with the cost of treatment, where treating a single patient may cost approximately around $10,000 per month, which is a major rise as compared to the $100 per month during 1960. This growth has brought along the huge cost of drug R&D (research & development) as well [6,8]. It is usually associated with a steep increase in the complexity of R&D process as observed in the last 20 years, which may be considered as a negative factor of the industry concentrating over highly composite disease and ever-increasing dependence. The ever increase in the demand of medicine has contributed to the wide diversification of the drug discovery approach in therapeutic areas, specifically cancer. Over the last 60 years, various strategies based on the varied biological as well as the molecular aspects of the neoplastic transformation have been used in pharmaceutical R&D [10,12]. This chapter mainly discusses the various strategies of drug design and development, where the major focus is over the various Swarm intelligence and the evolutionary algorithms conceptualized and proposed for the development of drugs and therapies related to cancer.

6.2 DRUG DESIGN AND DEVELOPMENT: PAST, PRESENT AND FUTURE

The whole procedure of drug design and discovery is extremely time consuming, heavy risk undertaking, and expensive affair, which takes about 15 years for the lead molecules to transform in order to approve the drugs [12,13]. The CADD (computer-aided drug design) has taken over as the most prominent tool in order to study and research the relation between the structure as well as the pharmacological properties of the chemical compounds as well as their adverse effects. CADD is majorly used in order to separate the most promising molecules from a set of large number of candidate molecules for the further experiment in the wet lab. The application aspects of the computational methods solve the purpose of identification as well as designing novel drugs since its advent in 1980 when the first report explaining the relation between specific psychochemical properties was published along with the potency of known inhibitors [1,14]. Since then for next 30 years CADD had a huge overall impact on the whole process of drug discovery [7,9]. The application of CADD in combination with high throughput synthesis, along with the screening, has given a heavy reduction in terms of both cost and time of drug discovery process—the computational methods which have themselves undergone a revolution at an immense pace. Many new as well as accurate ones are coming up since then in the same field as shown in Figure 6.1 [13].

The computational methods have been typically divided into two types:

1. Structure-Based Drug Design Method (SBDM)

2. Ligand-Based Drug Design Method (LBDD)

Structure-based: the concept of structure-based design depends upon the knowledge of the whole three-dimensional structure of the biological target achieved via methods like X-ray crystallography or NMR spectroscopy [15]. In the absence of an experimental structure for a target, a homology model can be created for the same based upon the experimental structure of the related protein. Using the structure of the

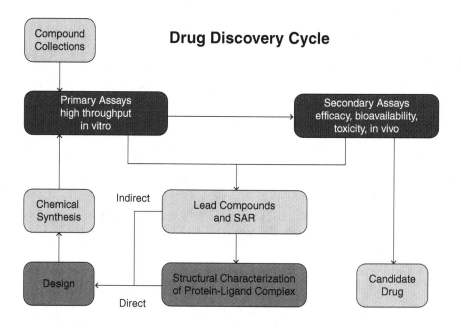

FIGURE. 6.1 Drug discovery cycle: ligand-based, structure-based drug design strategy [13].

biological target, the candidate drugs are predicted to bind with the high affinity and selectivity to the target that may be built using interactive graphics and intuition of the medicinal chemist. On the other hand, various automated computational procedures may be used to suggest new drug candidates [16,17]. The ongoing methods for a structure-based design can be roughly categorized into three main parts [18].

- The first method is about identifying new ligands for a given receptor by conducting a search over a large 3D structured database consisting of small molecules to look for the ones that fit the binding pocket of a receptor using fast approximate docking programs. This method is termed as *virtual screening*.

- The next category is de novo design of new ligands where the ligand molecules are built up within the constraints of the binding pocket by putting together either the small pieces in a stepwise fashion. These pieces can be either individual atoms or the molecular fragments. The main attraction of this method is its novel structure which is not contained in any database.

- The third method is the optimization of known ligands by means of evaluating the proposed analogues within the binding cavity [19].

Ligand-based drug design—also called as the indirect drug designing method, depends primarily over the knowledge of the other molecules that bind together with the biological target of interest. These molecules are generally used to derive a pharmacophore model that specifies the basic structural features a molecule needs to process in order to bind it with the target. On the other hand, QSAR model consists of a correlation existing between the calculated properties of their molecules and their experimentally determined biological activity may be derived. These QSAR relationships can be veiled in order to predict the activity of a new analogue [20,21].

Structure—Based Methods—generally used for the purpose of lead identification, e.g. pharmacophore development has played a major role in many of the lead discovery programs undertaken. An example of such method is docking-based virtual screening technique, while ligand-based methods are majorly used for quantitative structure activity relationships (QSAR) which is mostly being used for lead optimization [22,23].

With the introduction of high-performance computing concept (HPC) as well as modern parallel architecture in combination with the specific parallel programming models such as Open MP, Open CL, MPI and HPX, CADD and structure-based method have been implemented successfully in various drug discovery projects on a massive scale. This has enhanced the speed of the drug discovery project by the application of the heterogeneous systems that are equipped with various parallel computing devices [24]. The artificial screening process of huge database comprising compounds through the docking based vs. programs have been implicitly fast with the evolution of HPC where the computational cost has become quite cheaper comparatively. HPC also does allow the study of intricate molecular mechanism, e.g. allostery using computational methods which was previously unheard off [25].

The concept of molecular dynamics has then recently thereafter experimented in order to study more about allostery which happens to be a long-range micro-molecular mechanism of internal regulation [14,15]. This phenomenon was further investigated upon as well as studied deeply in order to gain vital therapeutic effects since particular kind of legends that are able to bind allosteric sites could be designed. From the drug design point of view, it is important to characterize the allosteric mechanisms behind the long-range interactions. These interactions are typically characterized by exploiting HPC as well as various accelerated approaches in order to perform simulations to be able to describe these mechanisms [26].

The blooming of HPC as well as soft computing techniques have provided solutions to various issues with extreme computational cost overhead, which were difficult to address upon previously. One of the prominent examples is problem of protein folding which comes under the ambit of structure-based drug design. It has been stated clearly and in an elaborative manner by various wide range application of SBDD that both HPCC and soft computing technique are responsible for bringing revolution in the field of drug design and discovery. However, not to ignore the fact that the number of successful applications of SBDD is few in comparison to the ones that have led to failure [27,28].

The failure of application may be accountable to many shortcomings of SBDD, in fact many can be reasoned out as due to the incorrect approach to the application of SBDD.

Keeping apart all these challenges and short comings, SBDD will definitely make a difference in future also. The continuous development as well as evolution in the areas of bio-chemical technology, software/ algorithms and hardware in combination would pace up the success range of SBDD in future [24].

6.3 ROLE OF SWARM INTELLIGENCE IN DRUG DESIGN AND DEVELOPMENT

The role of decision-making mainly comprises of searching through a large solution space. In the chemotherapy, one of the widely accepted cancer treatment, the size of solution space is increased exponentially with a number of participating decision variable whose value has to satisfy the feasibility criteria [28]. Here the criteria specified over the decision variables generally makes the solution spaces solution structure pretty intricate where the patches of feasible solution can be found scattered with only single region carrying the optimal solution. Here the major challenged faced in this process is obtaining a feasible solution for conventional optimization methods designed using gradient based simple heuristics [29].

Similarly, the method of mathematical programming may not be easily dealt due to the presence of multiple feasible regions in the solution space. Studies show that [27] Genetic Algorithm shows quite a good and robust performance when implemented over the class of non-linear, multi-constrained chemotherapy design problems. Nevertheless, field of evolutionary computation is growing where alternative techniques of computational optimization are being developed, one of the major concept is particle Swarm optimization (PSO), introduced by Kennedy and Eberhart [28].

PSO is a population-based optimization technique designed upon the socio-psychological tendency of the individual particles present in the Swarm, in order to immolate the success of other individuals [29]. The search behavior of particles is mainly dependent upon experience of its neighbors, which represents a type of Symbiotic Cooperative Algorithm, with a view to obtain an efficient search within the unpredictable solution spaces that have complex structure.

Equipped with the property of PSO may make method of drug designing particularly suitable to be implemented over the various optimization problem for chemotherapy as a treatment to cancer [30].

This methodology exhibits properties like multimodality, disjoint nature feasible regions in a solution space making the technique a unique approach to adopt.

Considering the medical aspects of chemotherapy drugs for cancer treatment, they all carry quite narrow therapeutic indices. This factor determines the dose level at which the drug consumption would have a significant impact over the tumor area almost reaching out to the values which may cause unacceptable toxic side effects. Hence more efficient treatments may result from balancing both the beneficial factors and the adverse effects as an outcome of combination of the various drugs administered in different dosages over a period of treatment [31]. The positive effects of the chemotherapy treatment here become the treatment objectives, which oncologist aim to achieve via administration of anticancer drug. A cancer chemotherapy treatment is carried out through following method [32]:

- Curative
- Palliative

Curative—This treatment is undertaken in order to eradicate the tumor.

Palliative—This treatment is chosen when a tumor tends to be incurable, and the goal is to maintain a reasonable quality of life for as long as possible.

The adverse impact of a cancer therapy stems from the systematic nature of its treatment, i.e. the drugs are delivered through the blood stream which affects all the body tissues.

As most anticancer drugs are highly toxic, they cause a great damage to all the sensitive tissues present at different positions in the body. As a means to lower this damage, the toxicity constraints have to be placed over the amount of drug applied during any given time interval on the basis of cumulative drug dosage over the treatment period as well as over the damage caused to the various sensitive tissues [33,34].

Adding to the toxicity constraints, the size of the tumor must be maintained below the lethal level during the entire period of treatment as a compulsory requirement for obvious medical grounds. In a nutshell, we can state that, the goal of chemotherapy is toward the achievement of the beneficial effects of the treatment objectives without going beyond the specified constraint variables.

The issue is well addressed by Particle Swarm Optimization where a set of variable schedules satisfying both the toxicity as well as the tumor size constraints yield an optimizing cancer chemotherapy in parallel humping intact the acceptable values of the treatment objectives [35]. The method allows the oncologist to come up with a decision regarding which treatment schedule should be used considering the preferences as well as the priority. A typical Particle Swarm Optimization problem is initialized with a population of random candidate solutions termed as particles [29]. These particles are thereafter moved through the hyperspace Ω of solutions available at the chemotherapy optimization problem. Here the position at each particle $(k + 1)_I c$ at iteration $k + 1$, corresponds to the treatment regimen of anticancer drugs where, k_{iv} is a randomized velocity vector, assigned to each particle in swarm. Here the velocity vector derives the whole of optimization process reflecting the socially exchanged information.

At this point, there can be a choice among three different algorithms that could regulate how the social information should be exchanged.

1. Individual best

2. Local best

3. Global best

Individual best—Here every single particle compares its current position in the solution space (Ω) to its own best position searched to this far. Here no information is considered from other particle.

Local Best—Here the particles take under consideration the best position within their neighborhood apart from their own past experience.

Global Best—Here the social knowledge used to affect the particles motion considers the position of the best particle from the entire swarm. Here each particle in swarms hence attracted toward the locations that represent the best chemotherapeutic treatment found by particles, neighbors or the whole population [28,29].

Based on this concept, various researchers have tried their intellect in coming up with the best optimized solution. Andrei Pelrovski, Bhawani Sudha and John McCall have proposed an article on optimizing cancer chemotherapy using PSO and GE Algorithm Concept [36]. There they have studied how various optimization algorithms and methods in PSO have been used to facilitate in finding chemotherapeutic treatments. It moreover performs an overall comparison with that of GE.

The field of Swarm Robotics inspired from the natural creatures and their social behavior has engineered minimal robots that use simple rules in order to interact with their neighbors and its local environment for providing a solution to the various complex real-world problems. Research scientists adopt iterative approach in order to design nano-particle treatments, injects them into a virtual tumor and improves their design till they reach out to a desired collective behavior. Once they obtain the nano-particle design, computer simulations as well as mathematical models may help to predict the cumulative behavior.

6.4 ROLE OF EVOLUTIONARY ALGORITHMS IN DRUG DESIGN AND DEVELOPMENT

As we know, designing a drug is all about researching as well as reaching a molecule that has certain activity over a given biological organism. A major portion of the effort while designing a drug is spent over trials in order to come to a conclusion whether the drug candidate meets the criteria of bio-availability, efficacy and safety. As it is desirable, a candidate should fail early in the ongoing trial process, rather being late. The pharmaceutical industry generally follows the ideal that fast failure is actually failing cheap. To fail fast and cheap, it is quite important to have fast as well as cheap methods of identifying whether the drug candidate carries the suitable properties in order to be drug or not [34].

The various phases of drug development are:

- Fine Lead Compounds: Use biological knowledge from genomics or proteomics to identify relevant drug target.

- Optimize Lead Compound: Test collection of compounds in cell based or similar essays and confirm activity.

- Perform Chemical Traits: Modify compounds to improve binding affinity and bio-availability to reduce toxicity.

- Identity Target Protein: Access whether compound is safe and effective.

- Market Drugs: Drugs are finally launched in the market [37].

One of the classes of methods that has been used in the pharmaceutical industry for this purpose is evolutionary algorithm, which is found to be typically apt for such purpose in an evolutionary algorithm, which is found to be quite appropriate as the drug design is largely survival of the fittest compounds.

In order to get hold of this lead compound for further drug design procedure, a set of compounds can be tested (called "libraries") for designing the biological activities.

A good library needs to have qualitativeness in efficiency as well as effectiveness. It should be small enough such that the list of testing incurred as lowest as possible, and so large such that the chances of finding a suitable lead compound are sufficiently high [37,38].

A rational and strategic selection of library contents enhances the efficiency as well as the effectiveness, since the compounds with similar structures undergo similar activities. A library carrying these compounds that are dissimilar in nature would need few compounds to search as much of the biological activity space.

Another criterion is drug likeliness, where the drug molecules must be having certain specific features. Such constraints can be enforced during the process of library designing.

With more information available such as structure, whether ligand or target receptor, where one would choose the compounds looking like target receptor looks like best fit rather into a more diverse one. This method is termed as "targeting" [39].

A common mode of constructing the compounds of the molecule libraries is combinatorial chemistry where a number of compounds belonging to group A having certain common reactive group in combination with compounds of group B having another common reactive group which may react with one of the reactive group in A.

Using this method, N+M reactants get converted into N*M products. A high dimension of synthesis (N+M+P regents may give N*M*P products), which can also be applied. Since there are many available reactants where multiple reaction steps can be applied, the number of potential compounds in comparison to the one which is practically as well as economically feasible in order to make and test upon. This make the selection of regents to be used quite a challenging task. This issue acted as a triggering factor that made use of evolutionary algorithms [37].

Many applications, algorithms as well as concepts have been presented in order to address this issue.

Gillet et al. [40] had an objective to construct a general library where the compound obtained had both traits of being diverse as well as drug like subsequently they formulated M_o Select [41], which aimed at finding a solution set such that for each solution no other solution in the set is equal or superior to it in all respects. The solution found was non-dominated or a perito-optimal.

Role of evolutional algorithms have moved over in order to find perito-optimal solution for some other context, which was quite a success, e.g. they were as efficient to get a set at a single run as founded by Deb [42]. Later, Sheridan [44] designed a combinatorial library of molecules built upon three fragments.

Apart from this Liu et al. [43] worked on same concept and generated two sets of compounds. Here first set was based on benzodiazepine template and the next one derived from (–) huperzine.

6.5 QSAR MODELLING USING SWARM INTELLIGENCE AND EVOLUTIONARY ALGORITHMS

The modelling of quantitative structure activity relationship (QSAR) was experimented for the first time by for imidazo, pyride and pyrazine, which makes together a class of phosphodiesterase 10A inhibitors. The PSO and GA performed the role of feature selection technique with an aim to figure out the most reliable molecular descriptors from a large pool [27,28].

Modelling off the relationships between the selected descriptors and the PIC_{50} activity data was achieved by the linear regression (MLR), the non-linear [locally weighted regression (LWR)] as well as the Mahalanobis M distances methods. Along with this, a stepwise MLR model was built using only limited number of quantum chemical descriptors that are selected due to their correlation with the PLC_{50}. Here the model was not found interesting. It was concluded with the LWR model, which was based on the Euclidian distance applied over the descriptors that were selected by PSO having the best prediction activity [45].

The QSAR modelling may be considered as one of the developed fields with respect to areas in drug development through computational chemistry. Similar kind of molecules with little change in aspects of its structure can show different biological traits altogether. This kind of relationship between molecular structures as well as the biological activities may be regarded as prime concentration factor of QSAR modelling [46]. The property predictions or any activity of interest have the capacity to save both time, money as well as minimize the usage of costly experimental designs, e.g. animal testing [47,48].

Hence QSAR model and QSPR models may be defined as the statistical models that are used in order to infer dependencies between the chemical structures, biological activities or psychochemical properties. The QSAR models are basically formed by mathematical functions that can connect the descriptors as well as the features generated out of certain small molecule structures to some predetermined activity or property curtained by experimental basis [17,49]. The structure activity study may show the traits of the given molecule that can correlate with some activity thus making it possible to synthesize new as well as more potent compounds that may enhance biological activities. The QSAR analysis based over the assumption that the behavior of the compounds may be correlated to their structure characteristics [50].

A QSAR model can be formulated as:

$$\text{Activity} = \beta_t + \sum_{t=1}^{n} \beta_t X_t \qquad \text{(i)}$$

where X_t is the set of computed properties of a compounds and β_j through β_t the calculated coefficient of the QSAR model [51]. The computational techniques are used in order to detect the functional group in compounds in the process of defining the drug discovery. This can be possibly performed using the QSAR which is comprised of the computation of every possible number that would describe a molecule rather performing a huge curve fit to search for the aspects of the molecule that correlates well the drug activity along with the severity of side effects [52].

The molecular parameters used for making an account for all electronic properties, hydrophobicity, steric effect as well as topology can be determined via experimenting practically or theoretically via computational chemistry [53,54].

The QSAR is typically used for the process of drug designing, discovery and development, and has a wide applicability for the process of correlating the molecular information with both biological activities and the psychochemical activities. Hence, the name quantitative structure property relationship (QSPR). The QSPR models have been often used to model as well as predict ADMET properties.

A QSAR model comprises [55,56]:

(i) QSAR Database

(ii) Descriptive Vectors

(iii) Machine Learning Approaches

(iv) Predictive model

(v) Validation

Particle Swarm Optimization—the concept of PSO was developed by Kennedy and Eberhart in the year 1995 based upon the social behavior of birds flocking or fish schooling etc. [28–30]. The principal concept of these population-based search techniques are based upon a group of living creatures that were randomly seen searching for food in the area, where each created is a particle contributing to the group in looking for the most favorable food.

In PSO, the position of the particle i in a D-Dimensional search space at time t, $X_i(t)$, is shown by

$$X_i(t) = (X_{i1}(t), X_{i2}(t), \ldots, X_{iD}(t))$$

Velocity (V_i), the particle is modified from its position to the current position is shown as:

$V_i = (V_{i1}, V_{i2}, \ldots, V_{iD})[19]$

The velocity vector of the particles flying from one position to other is optimized with respect to both particles' experience-based knowledge collected by social exchange of information from neighbors [18].

The velocity as well as the position can be calculated for each particle based on the following formulae:

$$V_{id}^{new}(t+1) = w.V_{id}^{old}(t) + C_1.rand(pbest_{id} - X_{id}(t)) +$$
$$c_2.Ran_d\,(gbest_{id} - X_{id}(t)) \tag{ii}$$
$$X_{id}^{new}(t+1) = X_{id}^{old}(t) + V_{id}^{new}(t+1)$$

where i is the index of the particles and d is index of position of the particle.

Rand$_d$ and rand$_d$ are the random values that range from [0, 1] sampled from uniform distribution. C_1 and C_2 are the acceleration numbers (cognition and the social learning factors). The methodology can be correlated to the QSAR model where the positions are defined in N-dimensional space, n representing the number of variables [54]. Here each particle has an associated value of the objective function (PLS or MLR error) depending upon the position. The particles here move according to the PSO rules, which define the new velocity as well as the positions. The rules here change the position in the direction of lowering the objective function (PLS or MLR error). In the current mode, PLS or MLR error reduces, which means particles may tend to positions where the relevant variables have associated values near to 1 along with irrelevant variables close to 0.

Evolutionary Algorithms—As we know the evolutionary algorithms are techniques which use the adaptive methods and may be used for solving searching as well as the optimization problems that are designed based on the genetic process of the biological creatures. Over multiple generations, natural populations have evolved based on principles of natural selection and survival of the fittest. By following the procedure, evolutionary algorithms can come up with the solutions to the real-world problems if they have been encoded in a proper form. The evolutionary algorithm normally consists of the Genetic Algorithm Domain, Evolutionary Strategies, Evolutionary Programming, genetic programming and the learning classifier systems.

The Genetic Algorithm have been used in the feature selection for QSAR with a range of Learning Algorithms, e.g. ANN and connection weights [53, 38]. The applied Bayesian Regularised Genetic Neural Network (BRGNNs) and GA optimized SVMs to QSAR modelling in drug design.

The Evolutionary Algorithm strategies applied to de-novo drug (or ligand design) [56] is a trial mode to generate the ligands from scratch, which is based only upon the information about the pharmaceutical target site or known ligands.

6.6 PREDICTION OF MOLECULE ACTIVITY SWARM INTELLIGENCE AND EVOLUTIONARY ALGORITHMS

One of the major issues in the area of drug discovery is to design efficient drugs against cancer. The current drugs have their own limitations including side effects, high toxicity, drug resistance toward present anticancer medicines [1]. These challenges require a consistent requirement to improve the drug arsenal in order to fight against this deadly disease. The general drug discovery techniques such as experimental methods are both expensive as well as time consuming. Thus, there is a demand to develop in silico techniques for designing anticancer drugs [8].

Few attempts have been made in the past in order to develop the computational method to design as well as predict the anticancer molecules. Recently, various studies have been carried out for modelling the drug behavior against the multiple cancer cell lines using the different genomic features basing upon these.

Genomic data which includes the DNA copy number give expression, mutation, and methylation—the drug sensitivity can be predicted. Here either a single or a multiple gene feature predicts [9,11] the drug sensitivity. In spite of the advances in the genomics, modelling the behavior of many drugs also comes as a challenging task.

The QSAR-based models can be regarded as the other possible approach where the chemical features are used in order to predict inhibitors against specified cancer drug targets [53].

As stated previously, CADD is a unique concept of designing the new drug molecule with the aid of a computer program. The term de novo in Latin means "from the absolute scratch," i.e. absolutely new or from the very beginning. The DNDD is basically a combinatorial optimization technique with a hue chemical space as the problem space, from where the drug like molecules or the optimal solution needs to be derived [41].

The two basic methods used for the designing drug like molecules in DNDD are:

(1) Atom-based method—here the molecules are constructed in an atom by atom manner.

(2) Fragment-based method—here the small fragments are used as the building blocks for the construction of the molecule.

Here the fragment-based molecule construction method is used in order to call out DNDD.

To address the issue of predicting the molecular activity today, many computer science techniques have been used to model *QSTR* or *QSPR* and develop various programs that would accurately predict how chemical modification and activities are influenced by recent algorithms and technologies [41,56].

One of the commonly caused side effects from the cancer chemotherapy is chemotherapy-induced peripheral neuropathy (CIPN), which is quite a life debilitating causing enormous pain. The multifactorial as well as the poorly understood mechanisms of toxicity have paved way for the identification of novel treatment methods. The computational models of drug neurotoxicity can be implemented in the case of early drug discovery in order to screen, in case of a high-risk compounds which chases the safe drug candidates for further development methods.

The quantitative structure toxicity relationship (QSTR) models have been formulated for the purpose of predicting the incidence of PN. The model here has been developed using a manually curated library of 95 approved drugs. The molecular descriptors that are reactive to the incidence of PN were identified in order to provide insights into structural modifications to lessen the neurotoxicity. The incidence of PN was anticipated on the basis of 60 antineoplastic drug candidates which currently are under the clinical investigation [54].

Quantitative structure activity relationship (QSAR): the QSAR model as discussed earlier are basically the regression and the classification models that can be used in chemical and biological science and engineering. The QSAR regression models can be related to a group of "predictors" termed as variable "X" to the potency of the response variable "Y", during the process of classifying QSAR model it relates the predictor variables to a categorical value of the response variable.

In the QSAR modelling, the predictors are composed of physico-chemical properties, also known as theoretical molecular descriptors of chemicals. The QSAR response variables may be a biological activity conducted by the chemicals. The QSAR model is a brief description of the bonding between the chemical structures and biological activities in a dataset of chemicals. On the other hand, the QSAR model predicts the activities of a given new chemical [56]. Here the relative terms are QSPR in case where the chemical property is modelled as the response variable. The different attributes or the behavior of the chemical molecules have been investigated in the field of QSPR. Few examples describing the fact are quantitative structure chromatography relationships (QSCR), quantitative structure toxicity relationships (QSTRs), quantitative structure electrochemistry relationships (QSER) and quantitative structure biodegradability relationships (QSBRs). The biological activity here can be represented as a quantitative example for expressing the concentration of a substance needed to give a specific biological response on the other hand, when physico- chemical properties or the structures are expressed by numbers, we can find a mathematical relationships, or the quantitative structure activity relationship among them. The mathematical expression post validation can be employed to predict the modelled response of divergent chemical structures.

A QSAR form of a mathematical model [55,56]:

Activity: (physiochemical properties and/or structural properties + error)

The huge size of chemical search space of the chemical compound database along with the importance of the similarity measures to drug discovery are the prime factors in the cheminformatics research. The increased size of search space has increased exponentially the number of available features in the dataset.

Though feature selection has been used in many fields like classification, data mining and object recognition, and has proven to be effective in order to remove irrelevant and redundant feature in the dataset, one of the attractive modes of solving the feature selection problems is the swarm and the evolutionary algorithms method. The typical example of swarm techniques are algorithms based on fish, birds, fireflies, while Genetic Algorithm in particular from evolutionary computation techniques [27,57].

Though researchers have tried their hands in Genetic Algorithm to depict the molecular interaction in the drug designing, they are yet to experiment the swarm-based algorithms for the same, opening scope for the further research work.

Genetic Algorithm: Multiple researchers have proposed articles where GA has been used for the purpose of feature selection model optimization and combinatorial search for docking studies [27].

Few articles have stressed over the GA applications to the quantitative structure, activity relationships (QSAR) modelling in combination with regression and/or classification technique. As we know, GA are stochastic optimization methods that are basically governed by the biological evolution rules influenced by the evolutionary principles [28]. GA has the quality of investigating multiple possible solutions concurrently where each explores different regions in the parametric space [29]. Here pollution based on N number of individuals is created where each individual encodes a randomly selected subset of modelling space where the fitness cost of each individual in current genre is determined.

Here, parent selected over the scaled fitness scores yield a fraction of children for the next generation of crossover where rest is selected by mutation. Hence new generation carries the characteristics from its parents.

This routine is executed until satisfactory or a global optimum solution is obtained. GA is quite an attractive model serving the purpose of optimization in the process of drug discovery, where every problem is highly particular due to its lack of previous knowledge of the functional relationship, making the generalization quite a challenging work.

6.6.1 Particle Swarm Optimization

As mention in previous section, PSO is considered as a robust optimization method, designed based upon the movement and intelligence of animals in groups [26,28], such as behavior of birds in flocks or schools of fishes that passes on the information regarding the current food location. Here every particle participating adjusts on its pbest and gbest values where, pbest is the position of the best solution found by the previous particle and gbest is the global position of the best solution available. The value of gbest undergoes updates only when the particle's pbest gives a value nearby to its target. Here,

W = weight controlling the velocity in order to enhance the convergence rate.

c1 and c2 = acceleration coefficients

rand() = function that returns a random value between 0.0 and 1.0 in for determining the significance of pbest and gbest [27].

For appropriate descriptor selection, a roulette wheel selection is employed into the PSO algorithm by viewing the location vectors of the particles that are stored in $x[i][d]$. Here columns of descriptors belonging to every particle are considered as a binary number [28]. The method is iterated until the maximum amount of iterations is achieved. However, the concept of PSO is only capable of extracting relevant descriptors considering its gbest value obtained from the best particle.

Even after a list of relevant descriptors is extracted, the appropriate theory regarding the significance of the relevant descriptors is needed. This issue was addressed by using other methods for creating a prediction model. Jalali-Heravi and Parastar [58] have compiled a report based on QSAR study for anti-HIV-1 activity of HEPT derivatives implementing

PSO for the process of feature selection along with SVR in order to develop the model. PSO and genetic algorithm have been used as feature selection techniques for phosphor diesterase 10A inhibitors [30]. The relationship between the selected descriptors and the pIC50 activity data has been achieved by multiple linear regressions in addition to locally weighted regression methods. Few researchers like Wang et al. [59] have tried to incorporate PSO for descriptor selection into the partial least square (PLS) method to obtain QSAR/QSPR models.

6.7 CONCLUSION

The chapter consists of a brief description of the need to predict molecular activity in the process of drug designing and monitoring over a body. Thereafter, it has briefly discussed the evolution and growth of the drug designing in the post and also elaborates the future aspects to look forward as an outcome of future discoveries. The next section dealt with the role of swarm intelligence in the drug design as well as development process followed by evolutionary algorithms in the next section. In the later segments, the QSAR model has been discussed in context to cancer drug research. Finally, the chapter states the aspects of molecular activity prediction and the role of Swarm intelligence and evolutionary algorithms for the same.

REFERENCES

1. Smith, H. J., & Williams, H. J. (2002). *Textbook of drug design and discovery*. 11 new fetter lane, London, CRC press.
2. Ghasemi, F., Fassihi, A., Pérezh-Sánchez, H., & Mehri Dehnavi, A. (2017). The role of different sampling methods in improving biological activity prediction using deep belief network. *Journal of Computational Chemistry*, 38(4), 195–203.
3. Merz, Jr, K. M., Ringe, D., & Reynolds, C. H. (Eds.). (2010). *Drug design: structure-and ligand-based approaches*. UK, Cambridge University Press.
4. Fosgerau, K., & Hoffmann, T. (2015). Peptide therapeutics: current status and future directions. *Drug Discovery Today*, 20(1), 122–128.
5. Ciemny, M., Kurcinski, M., Kamel, K., Kolinski, A., Alam, N., Schueler-Furman, O., ... & Kmiecik, S. (2018). Protein–peptide docking: opportunities and challenges. *Drug Discovery Today*, 23(8), 1530–1537.
6. Shirai, H., Prades, C., Vita, R., Marcatili, P., Popovic, B., Xu, J., ... & Clark, D. (2014). Antibody informatics for drug discovery. *Biochimica et Biophysica Acta (bba)-Proteins and Proteomics*, 1844(11), 2002–2015.

7. Tollenaere, J. P. (1996). The role of structure-based ligand design and molecular modelling in drug discovery. *Pharmacy World and Science, 18* (2), 56–62.

8. Waring, M. J., Arrowsmith, J., Leach, A. R., Leeson, P. D., Mandrell, S., Owen, R. M., … & Wallace, O. (2015). An analysis of the attrition of drug candidates from four major pharmaceutical companies. *Nature Reviews Drug Discovery, 14*(7), 475.

9. Swinney, D. C. (2013). Phenotypic vs. target-based drug discovery for first-in-class medicines. *Clinical Pharmacology & Therapeutics, 93*(4), 299–301.

10. Sams-Dodd, F. (2013). Is poor research the cause of the declining productivity of the pharmaceutical industry? An industry in need of a paradigm shift. *Drug Discovery Today, 18*(5–6), 211–217.

11. Sams-Dodd, F. (2005). Target-based drug discovery: is something wrong? *Drug Discovery Today, 10*(2), 139–147.

12. Hopkins, A. L. (2008). Network pharmacology: the next paradigm in drug discovery. *Nature Chemical Biology, 4*(11), 682.

13. Overington, J. P., Al-Lazikani, B., & Hopkins, A. L. (2006). How many drug targets are there? *Nature Reviews Drug Discovery, 5*(12), 993.

14. Butcher, E. C. (2005). Can cell systems biology rescue drug discovery? *Nature Reviews Drug Discovery, 4*(6), 461.

15. Paul, S. M., Mytelka, D. S., Dunwiddie, C. T., Persinger, C. C., Munos, B. H., Lindborg, S. R., … & Schacht, A. L. (2010). How to improve R&D productivity: the pharmaceutical industry's grand challenge. *Nature Reviews Drug Discovery, 9*(3), 203.

16. Yu, H., & Adedoyin, A. (2003). ADME–Tox in drug discovery: integration of experimental and computational technologies. *Drug Discovery Today, 8* (18), 852–861.

17. Dixon, S. J., & Stockwell, B. R. (2009). Identifying druggable disease-modifying gene products. *Current Opinion in Chemical Biology, 13* (5–6), 549–555.

18. Imming, P., Sinning, C., & Meyer, A. (2006). Drugs, their targets and the nature and number of drug targets. *Nature Reviews Drug Discovery, 5* (10), 821.

19. Anderson, A. C. (2003). The process of structure-based drug design. *Chemistry & Biology, 10*(9), 787–797.

20. Recanatini, M., Bottegoni, G., & Cavalli, A. (2004). In silico antitarget screening. *Drug Discovery Today: Technologies, 1*(3), 209–215.

21. Wu-Pong, S., & Rojanasakul, Y. (Eds.). (2010). *Biopharmaceutical drug design and development*. Totowa, NJ, USA, Springer Science & Business Media.

22. Scomparin, A., Polyak, D., Krivitsky, A., & Satchi-Fainaro, R. (2015). Achieving successful delivery of oligonucleotides—From physico-chemical characterization to in vivo evaluation. *Biotechnology Advances, 33*(6), 1294–1309.

23. Stocks, M. (2013). The small molecule drug discovery process–from target selection to candidate selection. In: C. Ganellin Roy, Jefferis Stanley Roberts (eds). *Introduction to biological and small molecule drug research and development* (pp. 81–126). USA, Elsevier.

24. Agrafiotis, D. K. (2002). Multiobjective optimization of combinatorial libraries. *Journal of Cmputer-Aided Molecular Design*, 16(5–6), 335–356.

25. Back, T. (1996). *Evolutionary algorithms in theory and practice: evolution strategies, evolutionary programming, genetic algorithms.* NY, USA, Oxford university press.

26. Bäck, T., Fogel, D. B., & Michalewicz, Z. (1997). *Handbook of evolutionary computation.* Oxford University Press, Inc. New York, NY, USA, CRC Press.

27. Cho, S. J., & Hermsmeier, M. A. (2002). Genetic algorithm guided selection: variable selection and subset selection. *Journal of Chemical Information and Computer Sciences*, 42(4), 927–936.

28. Eberhart, R. C., Shi, Y., & Kennedy, J. (2001). *Swarm intelligence (Morgan Kaufmann series in evolutionary computation).* USA, Morgan Kaufmann Publishers.

29. Nayyar, A., Le, D. N., & Nguyen, N. G. (Eds.). (2018). *Advances in swarm intelligence for optimizing problems in computer science.* CRC Press.

30. Clark, D. E. (1999). *Evolutionary algorithms in molecular design.* John Wiley & Sons, Inc.

31. Clark, D. E., Jones, G., Willett, P., Kenny, P. W., & Glen, R. C. (1994). Pharmacophoric pattern matching in files of three-dimensional chemical structures: comparison of conformational-searching algorithms for flexible searching. *Journal of Chemical Information and Computer Sciences*, 34(1), 197–206.

32. Lipinski, C. A. (2004). Lead-and drug-like compounds: the rule-of-five revolution. *Drug Discovery Today: Technologies*, 1(4), 337–341.

33. Leeson, P. D., Davis, A. M., & Steele, J. (2004). Drug-like properties: guiding principles for design–or chemical prejudice? *Drug Discovery Today: Technologies*, 1(3), 189–195.

34. Li, A. P. (2005). Preclinical in vitro screening assays for drug-like properties. *Drug Discovery Today: Technologies*, 2(2), 179–185.

35. Hansch, C. (1969). Quantitative approach to biochemical structure-activity relationships. *Accounts of Chemical Research*, 2(8), 232–239.

36. Petrovski A., Sudha B., McCall J. (2004) Optimising Cancer Chemotherapy Using Particle Swarm Optimisation and Genetic Algorithms. In: Yao X. et al. (eds) Parallel Problem Solving from Nature - PPSN VIII. PPSN 2004. Lecture Notes in Computer Science, vol 3242. Springer, Berlin, Heidelberg.

37. Lameijer, E. W., Bäck, T., Kok, J. N., & Ijzerman, A. P. (2005). Evolutionary algorithms in drug design. *Natural Computing*, 4(3), 177–243.

38. Yee, L. C., & Wei, Y. C. (2012). Current modeling methods used in QSAR/QSPR. *Statistical modelling of molecular descriptors in QSAR/QSPR, 2,* 1–31.

39. Gertrudes, J. C., Maltarollo, V. G., Silva, R. A., Oliveira, P. R., Honorio, K. M., ... & Da Silva, A. B. F. (2012). Machine learning techniques and drug design. *Current Medicinal Chemistry, 19*(25), 4289–4297.

40. Gillet, V. J., Willett, P., Bradshaw, J., & Green, D. V. (1999). Selecting combinatorial libraries to optimize diversity and physical properties. *Journal of Chemical Information and Computer Sciences, 39*(1), 169–177.

41. Gillet, V. J., Khatib, W., Willett, P., Fleming, P. J., & Green, D. V. (2002). Combinatorial library design using a multiobjective genetic algorithm. *Journal of Chemical Information and Computer Sciences, 42*(2), 375–385.

42. Deb, K. (2001). *Multi-objective optimization using evolutionary algorithms.* Wiley, New York.

43. Liu, D., Jiang, H., Chen, K., & Ji, R. (1998). A new approach to design virtual combinatorial library with genetic algorithm based on 3D grid property. *Journal of Chemical Information and Computer Sciences, 38*(2), 233–242.

44. Sheridan, R. P., SanFeliciano, S. G., & Kearsley, S. K. (2000). Designing targeted libraries with genetic algorithms. *Journal of Molecular Graphics and Modelling, 18*(4–5), 320–334.

45. Byvatov, E., Fechner, U., Sadowski, J., & Schneider, G. (2003). Comparison of support vector machine and artificial neural network systems for drug/nondrug classification. *Journal of Chemical Information and Computer Sciences, 43*(6), 1882–1889.

46. Ceroni, A., Costa, F., & Frasconi, P. (2007). Classification of small molecules by two-and three-dimensional decomposition kernels. *Bioinformatics, 23*(16), 2038–2045.

47. Evgeniou, T., & Pontil, M. (2004, August). Regularized multi–task learning. In *Proceedings of the tenth ACM SIGKDD international conference on knowledge discovery and data mining* (pp. 109–117). ACM.

48. Gärtner, T. (2003). A survey of kernels for structured data. *ACM SIGKDD explorations newsletter, 5*(1), 49–58.

49. Karelson, M. (2000). *Molecular descriptors in QSAR/QSPR.* Wiley-Interscience, Hoboken.

50. Kashima, H., Tsuda, K., & Inokuchi, A. (2003). Marginalized kernels between labeled graphs. In *Proceedings of the 20th international conference on machine learning (ICML-03)* (pp. 321–328).

51. Malik, J., Soni, H., Singhai, S., & Pandey, H. (2013). QSAR - Application in Drug Design. *International Journal of Pharmaceutical Research & Allied Ssciences, 2*(1), 1–13.

52. Livingston, D. J. (1995). *Data analysis for chemists. applications to QSAR and chemical product design.* Washington D.C.

53. Dudek, A. Z., Arodz, T., & Gálvez, J. (2006). Computational methods in developing quantitative structure-activity relationships (QSAR): a review. *Combinatorial Chemistry & High Throughput Screening, 9*(3), 213–228.

54. Papa, E., Dearden, J. C., & Gramatica, P. (2007). Linear QSAR regression models for the prediction of bioconcentration factors by physicochemical properties and structural theoretical molecular descriptors. *Chemosphere*, *67*(2), 351–358.

55. Ibezim, E. C., Duchowicz, P. R., Ibezim, N. E., Mullen, L. M. A., Onyishi, I. V., Brown, S. A., ... & Castro, E. A. (2009). Computer-aided linear modeling employing QSAR for drug discovery. *Scientific Research and Essays*, *4*(13), 1559–1564.

56. Gillet, V. J. (2000). De novo molecular design. *Evolutionary Algorithms in Molecular Design*, *8*, 49–71.

57. Chen, H., Zhou, J., & Xie, G. (1998). PARM: a genetic evolved algorithm to predict bioactivity. *Journal of Chemical Information and Computer Sciences*, *38*(2), 243–250.

58. Jalali-Heravi, M., & Parastar, F. (2000). Use of artificial neural networks in a QSAR study of anti-HIV activity for a large group of HEPT derivatives. *Journal of chemical information and computer sciences*, *40*(1), 147–154.

59. Wang, Y., Huang, J. J., Zhou, N., Cao, D. S., Dong, J., & Li, H. X. (2015). Incorporating PLS model information into particle swarm optimization for descriptor selection in QSAR/QSPR. *Journal of Chemometrics*, *29*(12), 627–636.

Index

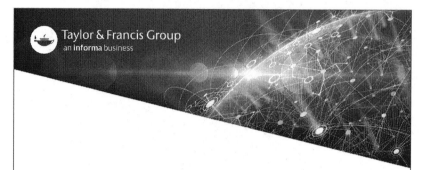